NKIJ'INEN TELUET

KINA'MATNEWE'L TELIMUKSI'KI WE'WKL ATUKWAQNN

KISI AMALWI'KMI'TIJ GERALD GLOADE

OUR GRANDMOTHERS' WORDS

TRADITIONAL STORIES FOR NURTURING

FEATURING THE ART OF GERALD GLOADE

PRUNE HARRIS, MURDENA MARSHALL, DIANA DENNY,
FLO YOUNG, SUSIE MARSHALL, CHERYL BARTLETT

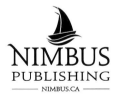

NIMBUS
PUBLISHING
— NIMBUS.CA —

Cape Breton University Press
Sydney, Nova Scotia

Kisikuk tle'k Mi'kma'ki alsutmi'tij wla 2013, 2022
Copyright 2013, 2022 Elders of Mi'kma'ki
Gerald Gloade art protected by copyright

Nimbus Publishing Limited
3660 Strawberry Hill Street, Halifax, NS, B3K 5A9
(902) 455-4286 nimbus.ca
NB1632

Weskijiwikasik kisi wikik/ Cover image: *Grandmother's Hands* (detail), Gerald Gloade
Kisi-tetk / Cover design: Cathy Maclean Design, Pleasant Bay, NS
Kisamko'toq / Layout: Mike Hunter, Port Hawkesbury and Sydney, NS
Kana'ta amkewes etliwikasikip / First printed in Canada

Responsibility for the research and permissions obtained for this publication rests with the authors. Mr. Gloade's art kindly provided by permission of the artist.

In addition, project funding support that made this book possible was provided by Cape Breton University's Canada Research Chair in Integrative Science Dr. Cheryl Bartlett and also the Atlantic Aboriginal Health Research Program (AAHRP) through the Canadian Institutes of Health Research— Institute for Aboriginal Peoples' Health. We would also like to acknowledge Barbara Sylliboy for her help with the Mi'kmaw editing and translation.

Library and Archives Canada Cataloguing in Publication

Title: Nkij'inen teluet : kina'matnewe'l telimuksi'ki we'wkl atukwaqnn / kisi amalwi'kmi'tij
    Gerald Gloade = Our grandmothers' words : traditional stories for nurturing / featuring
    the art of Gerald Gloade ; Prune Harris, Murdena Marshall, Diana Denny, Flo Young, Susie
    Marshall, Cheryl Bartlett.
Other titles: Our grandmothers' words : traditional stories for nurturing
Names: Harris, Prune, 1973- author. | Gloade, Gerald, illustrator.
Description: Written in English and in Mi'kmaq.
Identifiers: Canadiana 20210382678 | ISBN 9781774710869 (softcover)
Subjects: LCSH: Motherhood. | LCSH: Pregnancy. | LCSH: Mother and child. | LCSH: Mothers
    and daughters. | LCSH: Grandmothers. | LCSH: Grandparent and child. | CSH: First Nations—
    Canada—Social life and customs.
Classification: LCC HQ759 .H37 2022 | DDC 306.874/308997343—dc23

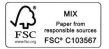 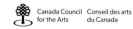 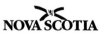

Nimbus Publishing acknowledges the financial support for its publishing activities from the Government of Canada, the Canada Council for the Arts, and from the Province of Nova Scotia. We are pleased to work in partnership with the Province of Nova Scotia to develop and promote our creative industries for the benefit of all Nova Scotians.

Nkij'inen teluet
Kina'matnewe'l telimuksi'ki we'wkl atukwaqnn

Our Grandmothers' words
Traditional Stories for Nurturing

Table of Contents

Table of Contents

NKIJ'INEN TELUET
KINA'MATNEWE'L TELɨMUKSI'KI WE'WKL ATUKWAQNN

Preface

TA'N MI'KMAQ TELI-KTLAMSITASULTIJIK WJIT KETU'-WUNIJANIMK

L'nu'k Ketlamsɨtasultijik poqji-kina'mat knijan teli-nqasayiw kejitu'n eskmalt mijua'ji'j, ula pkesikn wi'katikn wesku'tasik ta'n Kukumijinaq teli-ktlamsɨtasulti'tij wjit eskmalut mijua'ji'j aqq we'jitamk eykl kina'mu'ltal ta'n telkma'lsin aqq ma'w kikmaq ta'n tijiw mijua'jijk pma'ltj.

Ula wi'katikn maw-wikasikl klusuaqnn aqq kina'maqnn Prune Harris weja'tuajik newilijik Kisiku'k tleyawultiliji We'kwistoqnik. Teluisultijik Diana Denny, Murdena Marshall, Susie Marshall aqq Veronica (Flo) Young.

Murdena asukom te'silijik wunijink, newtiskeksijik jel ne'wijik wuji'jk, nanijik pitu'-wuji'jk aqq uklmuljin te'silijik wklniknk. Murdena wetapeksijik Muinaq aqq teliksua'lɨjik staqa wkwijual. Murdena teluet, "Tapu'kl koqoe'l mawi-ksite'tman ula wsitqamu'k. Maw-tumk ntli'sutim aqq ta'puewey Niskam."

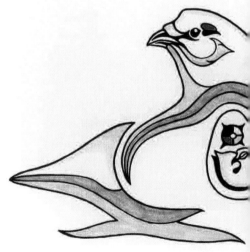

Diana tapusijik wunijink, nanijik wuji'jk, newtejilil pituwujijl aqq asukom te'silijik wklniknk. Diana mesnkɨs newtiska'q jel ta'puewey wtui'katikn newiska'q jel si'st tewije'kek. Kisikuis apaja'sijek kina'matnewey mɨta nutqwe'kek telta'sis mu nuta'q kina'matnewey mɨta msɨt koqoey ki's-kejitoq. Diana wetapeksijik Muinaq.

Susie newtiskeksijik jel tapusijik wunijink, asukom te'siskeksijik wuji'jk, tapuiskeksijik jel new'ijik pitu'-wuji'jk aqq newtiskeksijik jel ne'wt wklniknk. Susie na ketanaji waisisk aqq natawiteket, pu'taliewe'l kisitoql netui'skasikl msɨt tami wsitqamu'k. Susie wetapeksijik Jakejk.

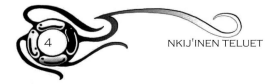

OUR GRANDMOTHERS' WORDS
TRADITIONAL STORIES FOR NURTURING

PREFACE

MI'KMAW WISDOM FOR PREGNANCY AND BIRTH

Traditional child raising practices recognize that you begin to raise a child from the moment you know you are pregnant; this book shares the Grandmothers' understandings for pregnancy and birth as well as some traditional stories that are used to help guide and nurture parents and children as they grow together.

This book WAs created by Prune Harris from the words and wisdom of four Grandmothers from the Mi'kmaw Nation of Eskasoni. They are Diana Denny, Murdena Marshall, Susie Marshall and Veronica (Flo) Young.

Murdena is a mother of 6, grandmother of 14, great-grandmother of 5 and godmother of 8. She is the Clan Mother of the Muin clan. She says, "I have two loves in the world. First and foremost is my language and second is my relationship with God."

Diana is a mother of 2, grandmother of 5, great-grandmother of 1 and godmother of 6. Diana graduated from high school when she was 43. She says she was educated late in life as she left school early because she knew everything! She is a member of the Muin clan.

Susie is a mother of 12, grandmother of 60, greatgrandmother of 24 and godmother of 11. Susie is a hunter and an excellent craftswoman, making baskets that sell far and wide. She is a member of the Lobster clan.

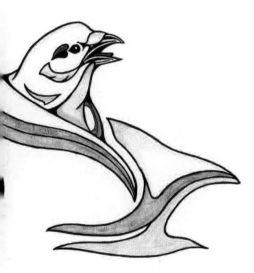

Willow Ptarmigan by Gerald Gloade (undated)

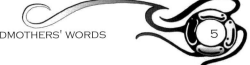

Flo newtiskeksijik jel ne'wijik wunijink, naniskeksijik jel ukmuljin te'sijik wuji'jk, naniskeksijik jel asukom te'sijik pitu'-wuji'jk aqq ne'silijik wklniknk. Flo na ketanaji waisisk aqq loqte'knikalajik aqq nuji-npiteket, ne'to'tk msɨt koqoey kiwto'qiw. Teluet "E'e, kesatm msɨt koqoey."

Prune tapusijik wunijink,t leyawip Cornwall, Eleke'wa'kik tujiw pejiwCsip Unama'kik, Elmiktaqamu'k. Naspit Integrative Science team CBU ta'n Cheryl Bartlett nujo'tk.

Cheryl na ekinamuet espi kinamatnoko'm CBU aq meki kisite'lmaji ta'n etkina'maji. Mawi ksatt alasij nipukuk tekwewa'j wikma, witapk aq nujikina'muaji aq maw wtu'emk lmujik ne'sijik. Ksatk ketkunij nipuktuk kisna pasik kwijimuk.

Gerald Gloade tleyawit Millbrook. Tapusijik wunijink, wel-nenut wjit tewji-nta' lukwatkl napuikasikl aqq elt panuijkatk ta'n wejiaq a'tukwaqnn Mi'kma'kik.

Aqq elt wela'luksiek Jane Meader, Mawpeltu wiki, wjit a'tukwaqnn teluisit "Ji'nm tleyawit tepknuset-iktuk." Jane nanijik wunijink aqq mekite'tasit nuji-kina'mewinu'skw aqq wjit teli-anko'tk kjijitaqn.

A'tuqaqnn wla kisi-wikasikl lnusikl toqo Mi'kmawis'sim mu tetuji nuta'wunn pikwelkl klu'suaqn staqa aklasiewiktuk.

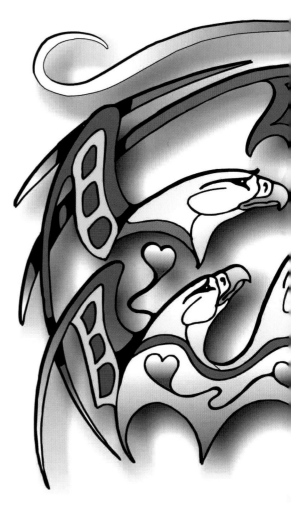

Eagle Family by Gerald Gloade (undated)

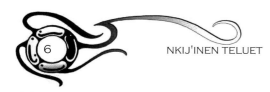

Flo is a mother of 14, grandmother of 58, great-grandmother of 56 and godmother of 3. She is a hunter, a trapper and a medicine woman with a keen interest in all around her. "Oh yes," she says, "I love everything."

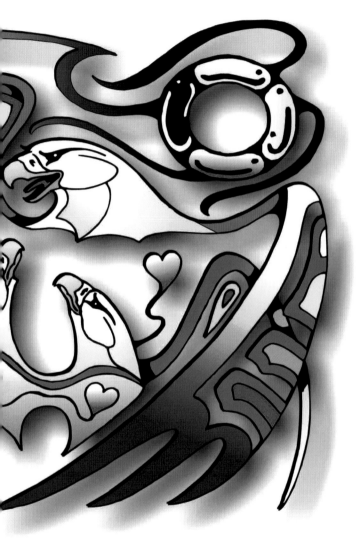

Prune is a mother of 2, originally from Cornwall, U.K., but now living in Cape Breton, Nova Scotia. She is a member of the Integrative Science team at Cape Breton University, directed by Dr. Cheryl Bartlett.

Cheryl pours her mother-love into countless students as a professor at Cape Breton University. She most cherishes being in nature camping with friends, family and her three dogs.

Gerald Gloade is from the Mi'kmaw Nation of Millbrook. Father of 2 children, he is widely acclaimed for his skills as an artist, as well as his passion for placing Mi'kmaw legends within the geographical landscape of Mi'kma'ki.

We are also most grateful to Jane Meader who lives in Membertou for the story of the Man in the Moon. Jane is the mother of 5 children and is a much-loved educator and wisdom keeper.

These are traditional Mi'kmaw stories translated into English. Mi'kmaw is both succinct and expressive and you will notice as you read these stories that there are many more words needed in the English telling. A single sentence of Mi'kmaw may require a whole paragraph in English. Equally, one word in Mi'kmaw can require a long sentence in English.

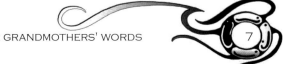

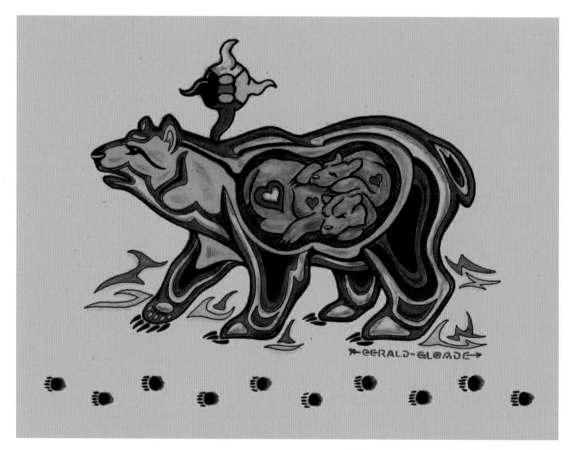

Twin Bears by Gerald Gloade (undated)

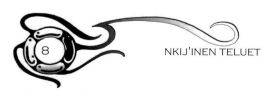

PROLOGUE

WELI-IKNMAKWEMK ~ TA'N TUJIW ESKMAQTMAMK

*S*ali'j na Mi'kmawi'skw. Melkiknat aqq weljesit. Welta'sit kesaljik wikmaq aqq welta'sit Mi'kmawin. Poqji-we'tuo'tk pilua'sik wtinin, mawi-amskwes apje'jk koqoey we'tuo'tk mi'soqo klapis pemi-aji-keknue'k. Na kejitoq eskmalatl mijua'ji'jl. Welta'sijik nekm aqq wji'numuml. Ela'tijik wkwijk, Wkiju'eml aqq Wkekkunitl. Ekinua'tuajik eskmalatl mijua'ji'jl. Welta'sultijik aqq wese'wiktua'titl.

Mawa'tu'tij ta'n nekmow tel-kina'makwi'tipnik wkwijua wejkwa'taqnik aqq ewe'mi'titl a'tukwaqnn kla'qij kina'muanew ula kjijitaqn Sali'jal. Na tel-kina'mua'tijik Mi'kmaq.

A'tukewa'titl Sali'jal kulaman kina'masilital aqq wle'tew teli-pkiji-skmaqtmaj. Sali'j tajike'tew wtinink, ta'n telita'sij, ta'n teljesit aqq wjijaqamijk mita kisiku'k kejitu'tij tajike'k e'pit na elp tajike'lital wunijan.

PROLOGUE

THE BLESSINGS OF LIFE ~ WHEN YOU ARE PREGNANT

*S*ali'j is a Mi'kmaw woman. She is strong, she is happy. Happy to be part of a loving family, happy to be Mi'kmaw. She begins to notice changes in her body, subtle at first, then more noticeable. She realizes that she is pregnant. She and her husband rejoice to think of welcoming a child into their lives. She goes to her Mother, to her Grandmother, to her Godmother. She tells them that she is pregnant. They hug her in joy.

They gather their knowledge and their wisdom from the teachings passed down, from women to women, over the generations; they share this knowledge, little by little, story by story. This is the Mi'kmaw way.

The Grandmothers tell these stories to nurture Sali'j so she can stay healthy throughout her pregnancy. Not only healthy in her body, but in her mind, in her emotions and in her spirit and they know that in this way the baby will be healthy too.

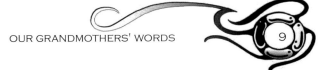

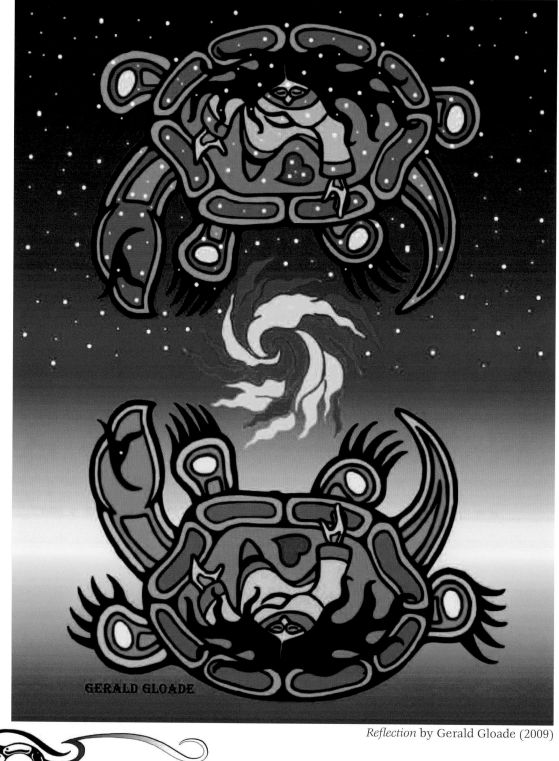

Reflection by Gerald Gloade (2009)

Msɨt wetapeksulti'k wsitqamu

Ni'n aqq Kiju' pemkopiek patawti-iktuk, etlelmiek. Kiju' telimit, "Kejitu'n katu kaqi-wasoqwa'sik ksiskw ta'n tujiw weskeweyin? Msɨt wen wetapeksit aqq wettaqne'wasit wsitqamu'k. Mukk elam wanta'siw kepmite'tmn wsitqamu, mɨta na'ku'set na kniskamijinu aqq tepknuset kukumijinu. E'pijik, wikmatulti'tijl tepknusetl mɨta nekm alsutk mimajuaqn, alsutk kjikapan aqq wasoqenikewuksi'k tepkik."

Na pipanimk, "Katu na'ku'set kiju'?"
Na telimit, "Kniskamijinaqi'k ne'kaw kejitu'tip na'ku'set ketmaqsɨteskikɨp Mi'kma'ki newtikiskɨk aqq nemitoqsɨp msɨt koqoey ta'n teliaq. Nemiapnik ta'n wenik tel-lukutijik aqq nekm newtukwa'lukwet kejitoq ta'n telo'lti'k, na wjit nekm kniskamijinu. Aqq ta'n tujiw poqnitpa'q elapa'timk musikiskɨtuk, nemiujik kloqoejk wasoqutijik, kejiu'kik na nekmow kjiknaminaq aqq kwe'ji'jinaq. Ne'kaw kelamuksi'kik, apoqnmuksi'kik aqq wasoqnikewuksi'kik. Ta'n tujiw kaqia'ti'k peji-nmiskuksitesnu aqq nikana'luksitesnu skɨte'kmujewawti eliaq wa'so'q. Mu elam newtukwa'lukutiwk ula wsitqamu'k, aqq ta'n tujiw wel-mikwite'tmn wettaqne'wasulti'k msɨt mimajuaqn, msɨt wen aqq msɨt koqoey, na tujiw mawi-ksasitesk."

Cosmic Connections

We are sitting around the table, my grandmother and I, laughing. "You know how much you shine when you laugh?" she asks me. "That is because each of us is related and connected to all of the universe. Remember to give great respect to the universe, for the Sun is our Grandfather, the Moon is our Grandmother. As women, we have a close relationship with our Grandmother Moon as she controls life, she controls the tides, she lights our way in the dark."

"And what of the Sun, Grandmother?"
"Our ancestors have always known that the Sun went through the entire country of the Mi'kmaq in one day, and saw everything that was going on. He saw what the people were doing, and he was the only one with this understanding, and that is why he is Niskamij, our Grandfather. And when we look up in the sky and see the stars shining in the dark, we know that they are our brothers and sisters, always watching down on us, sending us help and light. And when it is our time to pass on they come for us and guide our way as we walk the path of the spirits which we see in the sky as the Milky Way. We are never alone in this great universe, and when we remember how connected we are to all of life, to everyone and everything, then we are able to shine most brightly."

 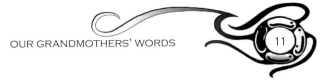

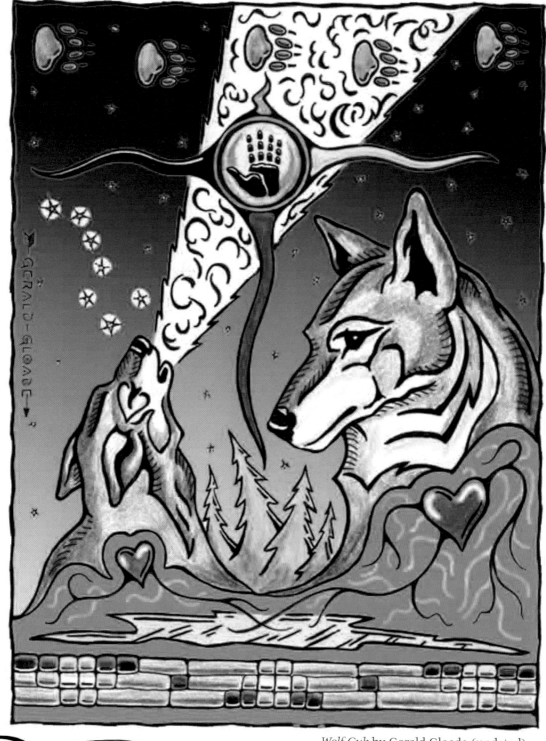

Wolf Cub by Gerald Gloade (undated)

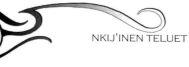

Wkiju'eml telimtl, "Pema'lit mijua'ji'j. Mi'kmaq teli-ktamsitasultijik mimajuaqn poqtamkiaq teli-nqase'k poqji-kitman. Ki's wjijaqamijl eymlitl mijua'ji'j. Nike' ki'l amuj menaqaj teleyin mita msit koqoey tela'teken kisna telita'sin we'tuo'tk knijan."

Mukk wkwayiw kisna i'mu ta'n wekayultijik kisna matn'tultijik, jel mukk ankaptmu amalapimk. Mita wkwayuti we'tuo'tew knijan aqq lue'witew nekm. Wkwayik wen, jiklapa'si kisna jikla'si ta'n eyk. Keknue'k ula wjit knijan wjijaqamijl.

Her Grandmother tells her "You have a life inside you now. For us Mi'kmaq, life begins at conception. Spirit has already entered that baby inside of you. And now, all your actions need to reflect that understanding. All your thoughts, all your actions, everything that you do you do to your baby."

You must not be angry, or witness any anger or violence. Not even on the television. If you do, then that anger will carry into your baby and he or she will be an angry child. If someone is angry, then look away or move into another room. It is of great importance for the spirit of the child.

Tapusijik Paqtɨsmk (kisna Paqtɨsm ta'n kesaluet)

Pemkopiek nuji'j. Newtiskekipuna't jel ta'pu. Newtiskeksijik jel ne'sijik nuji'jk aqq nanijik pitu'-nuji'jk aqq weljaqeyi. Ankamk nuji'j toqpiek. Nekm pilu'kaqnik wsitqamuem aqq ta'n telkaqnikɨp ni'n nutqweyanek. Ta'n tujiw ankamk nemitu ajipjutaqn, mlkikno'ti aqq kiskuk nemitu sespeta'sit; metu'kaqnik wsitqamu ta'n eymu'tijik knijjanaq kiskuk. Ankite'tman a'tukwaqnn wjit kikmanaqi'k aqq ta'n teli-ila'kwenuksi'kl ula a'tukwaqnn wejkwikweyanek. Mikwamit iloqamk na ankamit.

Pipanimit "Kujjinu, tal-kis-tla'sik pikwelkik eymu'tijik menaqaj telo'ltijik wenik ula wsitqamu'k aqq app pilue'k mu nestuo'lti'k, aqq mu ewlite'taqati'k aqq kesala'tikik wikmawaq?" Kejitu wkamlamunk wejiaq ula pipanikesit na

The Two Wolves

I am sitting with my grandson. He is 12 years old. I have 13 grandchildren and 5 greatgrandchildren and I live a rich life. I look at my grandson here beside me. In some ways he lives in a different world from the one that I grew up in. When I look at him I see hope, I see strength and today I see confusion; it is not always easy for our children who walk on Mother Earth at this time. I think of the stories, of the stories of my people and how the stories and the words gave shape to me as I grew. He sees me watching him and looks at me.

"Grandfather," he asks, "how come there are so many good people out there and then so many other people who are not good, who do not show any compassion or love?" I know this question is from deep within his heart

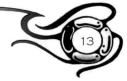

ankita'si ta'n tlimates. Ankite'tm ta'n tl-kinua'tuaq ula mijua'ji'j ta'n nsittew.

Na telimk, "Kwi's mimajuinu'k na pasik telo'ltijik."

"Mu apli'kmuj ankite'tmuk ta'n tle'tew, kejitoq amujpa ketaqma'sit aqq kamlamit, kejitoq amujpa kelamajik wunijink, jiko'teket aqq ketaqma'sit.

"Mu Coyote ankite'tmuk ta'n tle'tew, kejitoq amujpa tekweywajik wikmaq, ketanteket, altukwi'k aqq papit.

"Mu muin ankite'tmuk ta'n tle'tew, kesik nepat tujiw siwkw tukiet aji-ala'sin, alkusuen, mijisin aqq tkismin ke'sk mna'q app nepaq kesik ika'q.

"Waisisk mu ankite'tmuk ta'n tlo'ltitaq, kejitu'tij ta'n tla'taqatitaq aqq ta'n tl-mimajultitaq.

Na'sik mimajuinu'k amujpa ankite'tmi'tij ta'n ketu' tla'taqatijik. E'tasiw ala'tu'kl tapu'kl ankita'suaqnn ... tli-ankite'te'n staqa tapusijik paqtismk, newte'jit Paqtism menaqajewe'k aqq ktik Paqtism mu nestueyuk. Kitk ala'lu'kik aqq te'sikiskik matntijik."

Nuji'j ankite'tk ta'n kis-tlimk, tujiw klapis pipanimit;

"Ta'n tujiw paqtismk matnti'tij ... teken kespu'tuet?"

Na telimk, "Naqamasiaq nekmewey kwi's, kespu'tuet ta'n teken maliamt, ta'n teken mawi-eplew-smt. Maliamj pasik mu nestue'te'w paqtism na nekm ksipu'tuetew, maliamj pasik menaqajewe'te'w paqtism na wisuiknettew koqoey mu kelu'ktnuk etek kkamlamunk, mita menaqajewe'te'w Paqtism waju'et ksalsuti.

and I think to myself, "What message do I convey to this young fellow that will mean something to him?"

So I say, "You know son, only humans have this conflict."

"A rabbit does not have to think about how to act, he knows that he must eat and breathe, stay close to his family, be watchful, sleep.

"A coyote does not have to think about how to act, she lives with her pack, she hunts, she runs and she plays.

"A bear does not have to think about how to act, all winter he sleeps in his cave, waking in the spring to walk and climb, eat and swim, before sleeping again the next winter.

"Animals do not have to think how to act, they feel how they must be, and that is how they live.

"But humans have to think about how to act. There are two levels of consciousness within them ... let's call them two wolves; one is the good wolf and the other one is the bad wolf. They live inside each of us and are always fighting."

My grandson understands this; he thinks about it and after a while he says,

"If they are fighting ... who wins?"

So I tell him, "That is very simple, son; the one who wins is the one that you pay attention to more, the one that you feed the most. If you feed the negative wolf all the time that is the one who is going to win; if you feed the positive wolf then that one will overcome all the negative aspects of you, because the one thing that the good wolf has is love.

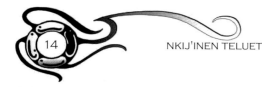

"Mu ala'tu'n ksalsuti, mu ksalsiwun, mu ksalawj kikma'j aqq mu ksatmu'n wsitqamu ta'n eymu'ti'k aqq mu ksalawj kniskamijinaqi'k aqq ta'nik wejkwita'jik na kis-wiswiknemuksitisk. Katu ala'tu'n ksalsuti na menaqajewe'te'w paqtism ma' elam wisuiknemat aqq staqa apli'kmuj, coyote aqq muin kjijitesk ta'n nuta'q tla'teken aqq na tle'tesk."

Telte'tm na wel-kina'muek ula a'tukwaqn.

"If you do not have love – love for yourself, love for others, love for the earth that you live in, love for the ones who have gone before you and the ones who are yet to come – then you can be defeated at anytime. But if you have this love then the good wolf will never be defeated and, like the rabbit, like the coyote, like the bear, you will feel how you must be, and that is how you will live."

I believe this is a wonderful story.

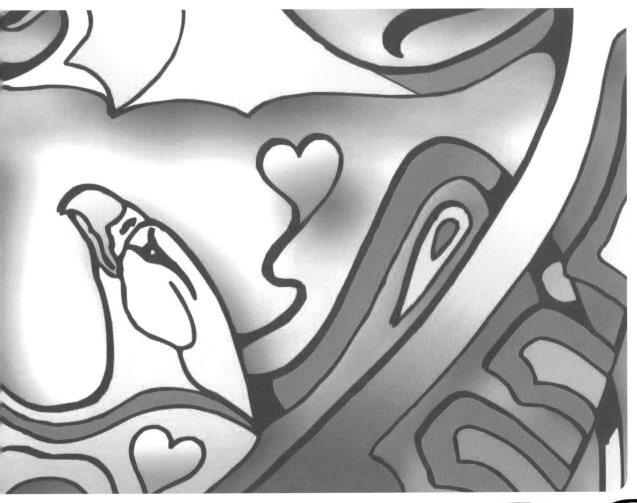

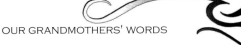

Ta'n tujiw Sali'j awsami-attikna'sit maliamaj wenik pilue'k, na wkwijl telimtl, "Amujpa na ki'l menaqaj teleyasin wjit na mijua'ji'j pema'lit. Kaqi-kispnulsin altukwi'mn maliamjik wenik pilue'k. Ajite'te'n maliamsin ki'l aqq knijan ke'sk mna'q al-pite'muewn."

When Sali'j is busy, rushing around to care for other people, her mother says to her, "Your responsibility is to take care of yourself so that you can take care of that baby inside you. Don't be a busybody or think that you have to be running around after people. Your responsibility to yourself and to your baby is far greater than to someone else who needs a cup of tea!"

APLI'KMUJ

Na' to'q wikijik Apli'kmuj aqq Wukumijl. Apli'kmuj na to'q male'k aqq Wukumijl amujpa telimtl koqoey nuta'q maliaptasin. Kaqnma'tij samqwan amujpa elulatl naji-nqana'pelin mita ma' skimtuk tla'tekek. Kaqnma'tij puksukl amujpa elulatl naji-esnoqnelin mita ma'

RABBIT

This is a story about Rabbit and his Grandmother, and in it, Rabbit is kind of lazy. He's not industrious and Grandmother always has to tell him everything that needs to be done. Grandmother has to say – when there is no water – she has to tell him, "Go get

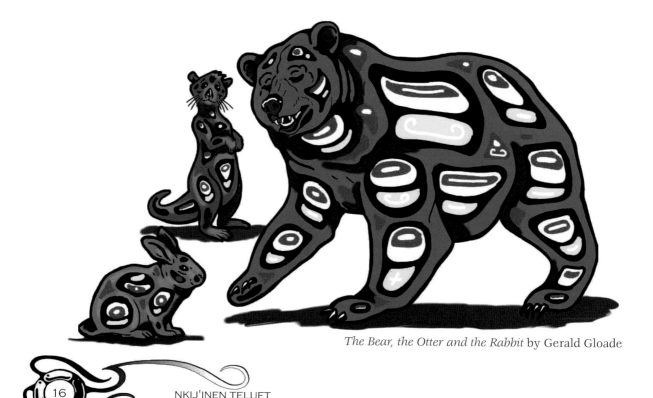

The Bear, the Otter and the Rabbit by Gerald Gloade

skimtuk tla'tekek. Mu nestuatpaq aqq pasik sespite'tk mijisimk, papimk aqq nepamk.

Jijuaqa na pisko'tal puksukl kisna naji-nqana'petew, na'sik maskite'tk attuklimk. L'pa mu kesatmuk eliet kisoqe'k naji-ktantun wela'kwewey.

Newte'jkek na'kwek, kesi-eksitpu'k Wukumijl telimtl, "Ke' pqoji-mittukwenej kiskuk. Ketu' naji-mittukwalk nitape'skw Muini'skw, wikit ala patatujk." Na Apli'kmuj aqq Wukumijl ilajijik tujiw semaqa'tijik naji-mittukwala'titl Muini'skwal aqq wuji'jl. Apli'kmuj aqq Muin welqatkik aqq papijik mi'soqo Muini'skw telimatl Muinal, "Kwi's kiskaja'tu wela'kwewey, smanej kikmanaq peji-mittukwejik." Muin telimatl Wukumijl, "Na kwesawa'l wow." Tujiw eliet a'se'k wiki'tij. Apli'kmuj kaqamit, iloqamatl ta'n tel-lukwelij aqq telita'sit, "Ketu' tal-lukwet apukwe." Mita Muin wessua'toq ki'kk waqn aqq mensikl ankoqsitann. Mawapja'sitl tujiw ela'tuatl wukumijl wissukwatmlin. Tujiw Apli'kmuj aqq Muin papijik mi'soqo kis-wissukwa'tij. Na epita'jik mijisultijik, malqutmi'tij wikk lasup. Apli'kmuj telita'sit "Naqamasiaq ula, kis-tla'tekek elt ni'n."

us some water," otherwise he wouldn't notice there was no water. And when the wood is depleted he has to be told, "Go get some wood, we have no wood." Rabbit does not see these needs on his own. He is irresponsible and only cares about eating, sleeping and having fun.

So, sometimes he will bring in wood, and make sure that Grandmother has enough water, but the one thing that he hates doing is getting them food to eat. He hates that he has to go into the woods and hunt something to cook for dinner. Something like a partridge.

One day early in the morning they get up, and Grandmmother says, "I think we'll go visiting today. I want to go see my friend who lives over here, to our left; we are going to visit the Bear Woman today." And so they get ready and leave to go and visit Grandmother Bear and her grandson. Rabbit and Bear play and they have all kinds of fun, and finally Grandmother Bear says, "Uh, Bear, fix something for dinner, fix something for our friends," and he says, "Well then, put the pot on. Make sure the pot is going well," and Bear goes to the back of the wikuom. Now Rabbit is standing there, and he watches him, thinking, "What is he doing?" because Bear takes the crooked knife from the wikuom wall, and he starts shaving his feet, shaving the bottom of his feet, like you do with calluses. Just like you do when you are making baskets, you shave the strip of wood, and you have little bundles of wood that fall to the floor, and this is what Bear did to his feet. Then he picked up the shavings and then he threw them in the bucket

Kisikui'skwaq emmitukwaltijik newtikiskik aqq l'pa'tujk papijik mi'soqo suel piskiaq. Na Apli'kmuj telimtl Wukumijl, "Amujpa elma'ti'k kwi's, poqji-piskiaq." Ke'sk mna'q elma'ti'k, Apli'kmujui'skw ankamatl witape'skwal aqq pipanimatl, "Ta'nuk naji-mittukwaliek katu ki'l?" Muini'skw ankita'sit tujiw teluet, "Pe'tapo'nuk sapo'nuk."

Mu awsami-pkije'nukek, Apli'kmuj Wukumijl telimtl, "Waqama'teke aqq msit koqoey wji-kaqi-maliapte'n." Tujiw pemkopa'sijik eskmala'tijik Muinal aqq

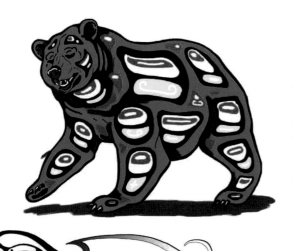

and his Grandmother took the bucket and washed them and threw them in the pot, and all the time Rabbit is wondering what is going on. He is thinking, "Why are they doing all of this?" But he went back outside with his friend and played until finally the Grandmother calls them, "C'mon boys, have your dinner. So they went back in and she served the tastiest soup in the world. Oh it was so tasty, and so easy to make. Oh, Rabbit couldn't wait to try and make a meal like this.

The Grandmothers were visiting all day and the boys were playing all day, and just before dusk Grandmother Rabbit told her grandson, "We have to go home, it's getting dark," but before they left the old Rabbit turned around and looked at the friend, Grandmother Bear, and she said, "By the way, when do you think you'll be coming to visit us?" And the Grandmother Bear is thinking and she says, "Sometime soon," and then the Rabbits go home.

One morning soon after, Grandmother tells Rabbit to clean the yard and straighten up and fix everything. She said, "Make sure everything is all set!" and then they sit down and wait for Grandmother Bear to visit. Finally they arrive and the old ladies are talking and playing waltis and the boys are playing and laughing. When the sun is high Grandmother Rabbit hollers to her grandson, "Bring the water in," and Rabbit remembers how Bear answered his grandmother and he asks, "Are you going to boil the pot?" and Grandmother says, "What? Why should I boil it? We don't have anything to cook. You haven't gone

Wukumijl pkisinnew. Klapis pekisinkik, na kisikui'skwaq aknutmajik aqq waltestajik aqq l'pa'tujk papijik aqq weskewe'kik. A'qatikiskik, Apli'kmuj Wukumijl telimtl "Naji-nqana'pe." Apli'kmuj mikwite'tk ta'n Muin telimapn Wukumijl na elp nekm teluet "Kwesawa'lit wow?" Na Wukumijl telimtl, "Koqoey wjit kwesawa'lates wow? Mu kiluiwk. Mna'q aptukliwun tujiw wlaku." Apli'kmuj telimatl, "Mukk sespite'tmu, ni'n maliaptites." Wesua'toq ki'kk waqn naji-musiksikl ankoqsitann staqa Muinal telamapnl tela'tekelij. Na wetnu'kwatk musiksmn wtankoqsitann. Ewle'jit Apli'kmuj, mu pase'nukl wtankoqsitann, na ta'n tujiw elayjitoq waqn wetewi aqiemtikaq, "Owwwww!" Sewisikek wkwatek.

Wukumijl nutatl na telita'sit, "Tala'teket nike'? L'pa na mu ankita'sik na Apli'kmuj." Na Apli'kmuj ali-aska'sit aqq altemit. Mal'tew altaqa'toq msaqtaqtuk, na a'ijkopilmuat wkwat. Na Apli'kmuj ali-aptu'sit, Wukumijl teluetl, "Ki's na nike' na'tuenaq telamasnaq, kesatk wet-napukwalaj wenik. Mu elam skimtuk kisi-te'tmuk koqoey nekm."

Na na'kwekl pemiaql, Apli'kmuj elisink mu kisi-alliketuk wkwat, Klapis katu nijkik na'sik mu puni-sku'tmuk Apli'kmuj ta'n tetuji-kejimkwaq me' wkwat. Wukumijl pemkopitl, mu talimkukl.

hunting since yesterday." But Rabbit answers, "Don't worry about that. I'll take care of it." Then he takes the knife from the wikuom wall, and he tries to do the same trick that his friend Bear had done to produce food for the pot; he tries to shave the food off his feet. But poor Rabbit, he doesn't have big pads on his feet like Bear. He has his foot on his knee and he is just going to shave it, but when he draws the knife through his foot he starts yelling Ahhhhh! Ahhhhh! Owwww! He had cut his foot.

Grandmother is standing there and she thinks, "What is wrong with him? Oh that rabbit, he only does things from somebody else's head; he never thinks for himself." So there is he, going around limping and yelling – there is blood on the floor, and they have to bundle up his foot. Now he's going around hopping with a stick, and Grandmother says, "Oh my gosh that rabbit! Can't he come up with any good ideas himself? Ever?"

Anyway, days go by and Rabbit is lying there with his foot sore, but finally he is able to stand up and after about a week he is able to take the bandage off and walk around, and in another few days he is walking along but of course complaining all through it. Saying just how sick he is, how sore he is, and how he can't do anything. His grandmother sits there, not saying anything.

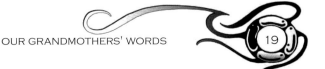

Klapis Nipk ika'q aqq Apli'kmuj kaqi-ila'sikek wkwatek. Newte'jk eksitpu'k wukumijl teluetl, "Ke' pqoji-mittukwenej kiskuk. Ketu' naji-mittukwalk nitape'skw Kiwniki'skw. Wikit inaqanek kikjuk sipuk."

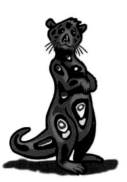

Na Apli'kmuj aqq Wukumijl ilajijik tujiw semaqa'tijik naji-mittukwala'titl Kiwniki'skwl aqq staqa L'nu'k, elt nekm tekweyatl wuji'jl. Apli'kmuj aqq Kiwnik welqatkik aqq papijik, wukumijuaq amal-aknutmajik aqq waltestajik. Poqji- piskiaq Kiwniki'skw telimatl wuji'jl, "Kwi's kiskaja'tu wela'kwewey, smanej kikmanaq peji-mittukwejik." Kiwnik telimatl Wukumijl, "Na kwesawa'l wow." Tujiw eliet sipuk, Apli'kmuj poqtukwalatl, ketu' kjijitoq ta'n tel-lukwelij. Kiwnik eliet sipuk tujiw kwetapiet. Klapis powkwija'sit, katewil oqlemitl. Eleketaq qasqe'k, tujiw ki's app kwetapiet, mu pekije'nuk powkwija'sit, ki's app katewil oqlemitl. Na Apli'kmuj jiko'teket aqq telita'sit, "Naqamasiaq ula, kis-tla'tekek elt ni'n." Na ta'n tujiw tepiejik kataq ne'pa'j Kiwnik apaji-l'ma'tijik aqq kisikui'skw wissukwat, katewapu'l eltoql. Wiklkik ti kataq. Ke'sk etlatalulti'tij Apli'kmuj

Some time passes. Now it is summertime and Rabbit's foot is all better. This morning, his Grandmother says, "I think today we'll go over and see my friend who lives over there on the right. We are going to visit Otter. So they leave the wikuom to see Otter and of course like all Mi'kmaw families, she has a grandson too. And the grandsons are playing and having fun, and the grandmothers are chit-chatting and playing waltes and having a wonderful day. As evening comes Grandmother Otter tells Kilnik, Kilnik the Otter, "Get something for supper will you?"

And so he says okay, and goes down to the shore; they all live by the shore. He goes down to the shore and, of course, Rabbit follows him and he sees what kilnik does. He dives from the bank of the river and goes into the water. It takes him a while to come up, but when he does, he has an eel in his mouth. He throws it to the ground, and then he does it again. He dives and is gone for a little while, and when he comes up he has another eel. All the while, Rabbit is watching and thinking, "Oh my goodness, this is even easier than how Bear got food! You don't have to hurt yourself at all." And he's watching the otter, and sees that soon Otter has a string of eels. And they take them up to the wikuom and of course the old lady cooks – the pot was already boiling and she starts to make eel stew. And oh! what a supper they had. It is summer, the evenings are long, and oh! what a wonderful, delicious meal. And all the time he is eating, Rabbit is thinking, "This is even easier than what happened

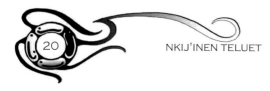

ankita'sit, "Naqamasiaq ula tel-tuklimk, wetnu'kwatm na."

Mu awsami-pkije'nukek, Apli'kmuj Wukumijl telimtl, "Waqama'teke aqq msit koqoey wji-kaqi-maliapte'n." Tujiw pemkopa'sijik eskmala'tijik Kiwnikal aqq Wukumijl pkisinnew. Welqatk ti Apli'kmuj, jel mu kis-wantaqpik, wkwatl etliaql, eskamalajik Kiwnikal aqq Wukumijl pkisinnew. Welqatmu'tijik, amal-aknutma'tijik aqq papultijik. Klapis Apli'kmuj Wukumijl wenaqa'sitl kiskaja'tun wela'kwewey. Poqji-wsawa'laj wowl, Apli'kmuj weji-wunaqsink telimatl, "Mukk samatu koqoey ni'n maliaptites wela'kwewey. Epukjik pkisitutes." Apli'kmuj wet-napikwalatl Kiwnikal. Eli'pit sipuk tujiw kwetapiet. Na mu apaji-powkwija'sikaq! Kiwnik elapit, eskmalatl powkwija'silin katu mu tela'sinuk! Mita mu Apli'kmuj natawi'kweyuk! Mu apli'kmuj natawi'kwolti'k aqq mu natawi-wktapia'ti'k. Kiwnik poqji-sespeta'sit. Klapis paqasu'naqiet aqq natqayjimatl Apli'kmujl.

Elisma'latl qasqe'k tujiw apaji-minu'natl, Apli'kmuj wukumijl kaqi-nmitoq ta'n teliaq, na pepueket wun'ji. Telita'sit, "Ki's app! Ki's na nike' na'tuenaq telamasnaq. Suel kwetapa't ke'sk kaqasi-mila'tekej."

Na Kiwnik elma'latl Apli'kmujl. Apli'kmuj kispnet, piskwapekit aqq epasma'sit. Weloqatalulti'tij wikmaq, nekm mu mijisik siawi- awni'skwesink, kewjit aqq netakeyasit. Welta'sit me' mimajit. Wukumijl telimatl, "Mu keju'lnu kwi's, kaqasi-mila'teken. Mu kejitu nuku' ta'n tla'lultes."

the other day, I want to try getting our food like this."

A few days go by and Grandmother announces that her friend Otter is coming today, and she asks that Rabbit clean the yard and straighten up and fix everything. She says, "Make sure everything is all set!" and then they sit down and wait for Grandmother Otter to visit. Rabbit is excited, so he's sitting there with his legs moving and he can't wait for the old lady to come and bring her grandson to play. And what a day they have, playing and talking. Later on, Grandmother Rabbit wants to cook something for dinner. When she goes to get up to get some water on, Rabbit jumps in and he says, "No! Don't touch anything. I'll bring supper in a minute." Now what do you think he does? Of course he tries to do the same thing he saw Otter doing. He goes to the shore and he dives right in. The problem is, he never comes up! Otter is waiting for him to come up and he isn't coming up! Because Rabbits can't swim!

He doesn't know how to swim, and rabbits don't swim, and they don't know how to dive, so he is gone for a little while and Otter is getting nervous, until he can't stand it anymore and he jumps in and hauls Rabbit out.

He brings him to the shore and revives him, and meanwhile, the old lady is standing there shaking her head. "He did it again! Where he learned that trick, I don't know, but it practically killed him. And of course after he is revived, he is exhausted. He just crawls up to the wikuom and lies down. I don't know what the old lady cooks for supper

Newtipunqek pemiaq, Apli'kmuj me' pemi-ntake'k ta'n telitpiep. Siwkw ika'q aqq welikiskik, wukumijl teluetl, "Ke' pqoji-mittukwenej kiskuk. Ketu' naji-mittukwalk nitape'skw Apo'qejiti'skw. Mu ela'tiwk sipuk aqq mu menuaqalnu kaqasi-mila'teken. Mu ela'tiwk patatujk kisna inaqanek mita na'te'l jileyu'tip. Kiskuk pektaqa'si'k wikij Apo'qejiti'skw. Na Apli'kmuj aqq Wukumijl ilajijik tujiw semaqa'tijik naji-mittukwala'titl Apo'qejiti'skwl aqq wuji'jl. Welqatmu'tijik, kisikui'skwaq aknutmajik aqq l'pa'tujk papijik aqq weskewe'kik. Klapis suel piskiaq, Apo'qejit wukumijl pipanimatl, "Api-ktansipnik juji'jk sepay?"

that night, but Rabbit is cold and under the covers and embarrassed, and he has no supper, and he is just thankful to be alive, and Grandmother Rabbit says, "I don't know Rabbit, you do such crazy things, I don't know what to do with you."

A year goes by. Rabbit is still embarrassed from his ordeal, but it is spring, a nice spring morning, and Grandmother says, "We are going to visit my friend, the Woodpecker. And we're not going near water, and I don't want you to do anything daft. We're not going to the left because you got hurt after going that way, and we are not going to the right because you got hurt after you went that way. So what we are going to do this day is to go straight up, over there. Woodpecker doesn't live far, and today we'll visit them." And so they go. Grandmother Woodpecker is so glad to see her friend and they spend the day chit-chatting and doing all kinds of things, and the boys are playing and laughing, until close to evening time when Grandmother Woodpecker calls out to her grandson, "Did you collect fresh bugs this morning?"

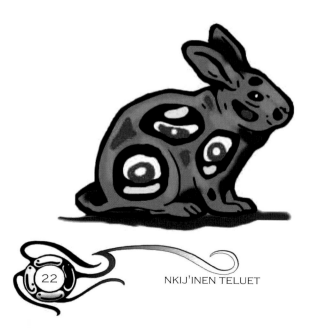

Apo'qejit teluet, "Meskeyi, awanta'sias, naji-ktankik nike'." Na ankmayiw semaqa'sit. Eliet kaqamitl meskilkl kmu'jl aqq so'qiet aqq poqji-matta'tl kmu'jl ewe'wk wsisqun. Ankmayiw we'jiajik pikwelkik aqq milamuksijik jujijk aqq pitkmalajik eptaqn-iktuk. Apo'qejit niskusua't aqq elma'tuajik jujijk wukumijl wissukwalan. Apli'kmuj teli-pkiji-jikeywatl ta'n tel-lukwelij, na nike' telita'sit, "Naqamasiaq ula tel-tuklimk! Ma' wktapa'w aqq ma' sewissmuan nkatl, wetnu'kwatm na."

Ke'sk mna'q elma'ti'k Apli'kmujui'skw ankamatl witape'skwal aqq pipanimatl, "Ta'nuk naji-mittukwaliek katu ki'l?" Apo'qejiti'skw ankita'sit tujiw teluet, "Pe'tapo'nuk sapo'nuk." Na te'sikiskik Apli'kmuj aqq Wukumijl eskinuapijik, eskmala'tijik Apo'qejitl aqq Wukumijl peji-mittukwenew. Klapis pekisinlijik. Newtikiskik l'pa'tujk welqatkik papijik aqq alkusuejik. Klapis Apli'kmujui'skw wenaqa'sit naji-kiskaja'toq wela'kwewey, Apli'kmuj weji-wenaqsink telimatl, "Ke' ni'n maliaptmap wela'kwewey." Aqq tewietaq. Eliet kaqamitl meskilkl kmu'jl aqq so'qiet aqq pasik kis-lekejek wun'jiek aqq pem-nisietaq. Mal'tewiaq wsisqun elisink petkwe'k. Apli'kmujui'skw tel-ne'a'sit nemiatl. Pepueket wun'ji aqq teluet, "Ki's app! Ki's na nike' na'tuenaq telamasnaq. L'pa mu nsituo'qnmik na Apli'kmuj!"

Woodpecker replies, "Oh! I forgot, I'll go and get some now." And straight away he goes and climbs up the tree where he starts pounding on the tree with his long beak: tap tap tap! Quickly, he gets a lot of bugs, of different kinds of bugs that are up there, and as he gets them he puts them in the basket: tap tap tap tap! Before too long the basket is halfway full. Woodpecker comes down from the tree and his Grandmother makes the most beautiful meal out of the bugs. And who do you think watched Woodpecker getting the bugs? Rabbit! And now Rabbit is thinking, "Well, this is even easier. You don't have to drown, you don't have to cut your feet; this is the easiest trick of all. I am going to try it."

Before Rabbit and his Grandmother leave they ask Grandmother Woodpecker when she would come and visit them. "Oh, a little later on in the spring I'll come and visit you." So every day in the spring Rabbit and his Grandmother wait, and putter around and keep the place tidy and finally a day arrives when Grandmother Woodpecker arrives with her grandson. All day the two boys play, climbing and running and having great fun. Finally when Grandmother wants to fix supper, Rabbit leaps up and says, "Don't do anything yet; I'll bring home supper in a second." So he goes up the tree and gets ready and then: tap tap tap! He bangs his head on the tree and zzzzzzbam! With a bloody nose, he slides down the tree, right down to the ground, and lies there, out like a light. From the first bang of his head he is unconscious.

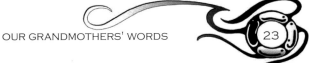

Elmiketna'titl aqq kasikwo'tla'titl aqq tekpa'q elo'tua'tij, na klapis katu tukwatpa't. Paqsipki-ntakeyasit na piskwapekit aqq epasma'sit, anquna'toq wun'ji aqq ankita'sit. Ta'n tujiw Wukumijl piskwa'lij kne'ji'jk telimatl, "Kiju' elui'tmasi mu lutuan pilue'k waisisk ta'n tel-kwilmi'tij wilu'ew. Nike' weja'tekemk ankita'sites aqq kisita'sites ta'n tl-kwiltes kilu'nu." Wukumijl telimtl, "Na kwi's nike' tetpaqita'sin!"

And the old lady comes out and says, "Oh my goodness, he did it again! Where does he come up with these ideas? He is crazy." So they carry him home and put cold water on his head and they clean his bloody nose and finally he wakes up. Of course he's embarrassed and he crawls to his bed and he hides his head and thinks to himself. When his Grandmother comes in later, he speaks to her, "Kiju, from now on, I'm going to think for myself and come up with my own ideas." And his Grandmother looks at him and says, "Grandson, I think that is the best idea that you have had!"

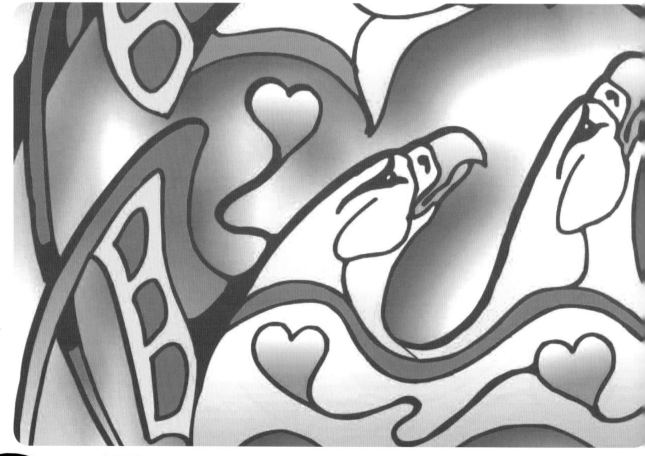

HEWEY HEADLEY

Ula na Niskamijinenaq a'tukwaqnm. Tleyawitaq Ktaqamkuk aqq newte'jkek ji'nmuk wtlukwaqnuewek na esnoqna'tinew wjit wikmawaq. Na meski'kek aqq kelu'kek nipukt eteksipnek kikjuk L'nue'katik ta'n L'nu'k ne'kaw etli-esnoqna'tisnik. Menaqewo'tmekip, mu musikte'muek pasik wesua'tuek tepiaq kmu'j wi'ka'tinen aqq mawse'nmanen, aqq pasik temasqite'kitjik kmu'jk ta'n tel-nuta'iek. Welo'tmekip nipukt aqq nipukt weleyuksiekip. Na, Kajjimen wejiet Qame'k pekwatelkisnek ula maqamikewek aqq pejiwsis naji-wikin nmaqamikewminen. Eykipnik pilue'k Kajjimenaq wejuowk L'nue'kati keltituetu'tij kmu'j. Hewey Headley teluisit mawi-knat aqq mawi-mqe'k Kajjimen katu na Kajjimen ta'n kistelkip maqamikew kikjuk L'nue'katik elt maqe'k.

Ta'n tujiw nemiaj L'nu'l kikjuk wmaqamikem, poqtiteskuatl aqq ketu' pe'skuatl. Niskamijinen aqq ktikik ji'nmuk kisa'matultijik ma' esnoqna'ti'k ula ji'nml wmaqamikemk mita awsami-maqe'kl, na Niskamij alimknkl kmu'ji'jl aqq psetkunn ta'n nisputuatkl wju'sn. Na newte'jkek na'kwek, Niskamij nutmat nepilitaq ula Kajjimenaq. Na ji'nmuk kisita'sultijik apajita'new na maqamikew ta'n i' tli-esnoqna'tisnik. Mawa'lsultijik ji'nmuk aqq naji- esnoqna'tijik.

HEWEY HEADLEY

This is one of our grandfather's stories. He is from Newfoundland and one of the jobs that the men do is to cut logs for the needs of the community. Now there is a big, beautiful wood close to the reserve that we Mi'kmaq have always been able to cut wood from. Respectfully, not clear cutting, but taking some wood for what we need for building and firewood, and taking only the trees that it is okay to take. We care for the wood and the wood cares for us. Well, this wood gets bought by a man from Scotland who comes over to live on our land. There are several Scottish men in the area and, of course, they don't want us to be cutting down trees in "their" woods. Hewey Headley is the meanest and strongest of all the Scots, but the one that bought the wood close to the reserve. He is pretty mean too.

If he sees a Mi'kmaw man near his property he chases him away with a shotgun. Our grandfather and the other men decide that they will not even cut one stick of wood from his land because of his meanness, so Grandfather spends a lot of his time collecting twigs and branches that have fallen in the winds. But one day, Grandfather hears that the Scotsman has died. The men meet and decide that some of them they will go into the woods that have always provided for us and cut some hardwood. So a group goes to get the hardwood, happy to be back in the trees that they have known all their life.

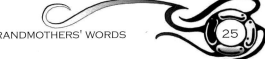

Tema'kipula'titl newte'jilitl kmu'jl, tujiw app ktikl, ke'sk etl-lukuti'tij amal-aknutma'tijik aqq weskewo'ltijik, na si'stewe'l kmu'jl poqji-tema'kipula'tij nutua'titl na'tuenl knekk wetewisawetl,

"Wen eyk? Wen net ki'l?"

L'nu'k telta'sultijik paqtoqewa'q kisna wju'sn nutmi'tij. Na siaw-lukutijik.

Na'sik ki's app nutua'tijl na'tuenl wetewisawetl,

"Wen eyk? Wen net ki'l?"

Nike' aji-wejuow metewa'toq, L'nu'k alapetesultijik. Newte'jit teluet, "Etuk jel na Kajjimeno'q?" Ktikik telua'tijik, "Mu na nekm, nepkipnaq."

Ki's app si'stewey nutua'tijl na'tuenl "Wen eyk? Wen net ki'l?"

Aji-wejuow nike' wetewisawetl. Telsitua'titl ala ktuatqituk i'mlin, na ji'nmuk wesimkutijik, elmitukwi'multijik wutanmuaq. Ika'tij wutank, elta'titl Niskamijl aqq aknutmua'titl ta'n kis-tlitpio'lti'tij. Telima'titl Kajjimenaq wskite'mujml eymlitl kisoqe'k aqq me' keltituet maqamikew, ma' kisi-naji-esnoqna'ti'k na'te'l.

Niskamij ankita'sit tujiw telimajik, "Jukwita'q! Apajita'nej kisoqe'k. Naji-esnoqna'ti'k." Na poqtamkita'jik, Niskamij nikana'sit. Ji'nmuk me' we'kwata'sultijik, wtejk wetukwala'titl. Ika'tij ta'n etli-esnoqna'tipnik aqq poqji-tma'kittaqatijik. Ankmayiw nutua'titl Kajjimenl kesikawa'tulitl,

"Wen eyk? Wen net ki'l?"

Tewji-wjuowk wetsitua'titl, jel alapetesultijik, eskmala'titl

They cut one log. They cut another log. The men are talking and laughing, but as they cut a third log they hear a voice, calling from a distance,

WHO IS THERE? WHO ARE YOU?

And the Mi'kmaw men think, "Oh it's only an echo, or maybe the wind." And they keep on cutting wood.

But pretty soon they hear the voice again,

WHO IS THERE? WHO ARE YOU?

This time it is closer, and the men look around them nervously. "Is it him? Is it the Scottish man?" one of them says. But they say to each other, "Aahh it's nobody, it can't be him, he died."

But a third time someone hollers, WHO IS THERE? WHO ARE YOU?

And this time the voice is very close. It sounds like it is just behind these bushes and all the men take off, running back to the reserve as fast as they can. When they get there, they rush up to our Grandfather and tell him what has happened. They tell him that the ghost of the mean Scot is still in the woods and that they still aren't able to cut any hardwood.

So Grandfather thinks and then says, "Come on! Let's go back to the wood. We are going to get those logs." And he confidently starts striding away with the other men following, still a bit afraid. They get to the fallen logs and start cutting. Within minutes they hear the strong Scottish voice asking,

WHO IS THERE? WHO ARE YOU?

The voice is so close that the men are looking around expecting to see him standing there. But Grandfather stands

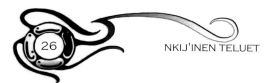

wejkupukuilin. Na Niskamij kaqamtesink aqq se'skwet, "Ni'n na Hewey Headley."

Wantaqteskek eymi'tij, l'pa mu mattenuk aqq mu wen me'tek. Klapis Niskamij aqq ji'nmuk nutua'titl na'tuenl, sankewa'toql, "A', weliaq." Aqq mu app lukwaqna'lukwi'tikaq Kajjimenaq.

up straight and loud as he can and shouts, "I am Hewey Headley."

For a long while there is silence in the woods. You could hear a pin drop. Silence in the woods as nobody and nothing stirred. Then, a few minutes later, from a long way off in the distance Grandfather and the men hear a soft voice say, "Och aye! That's okay, then," and they were never bothered by that Scotsman again.

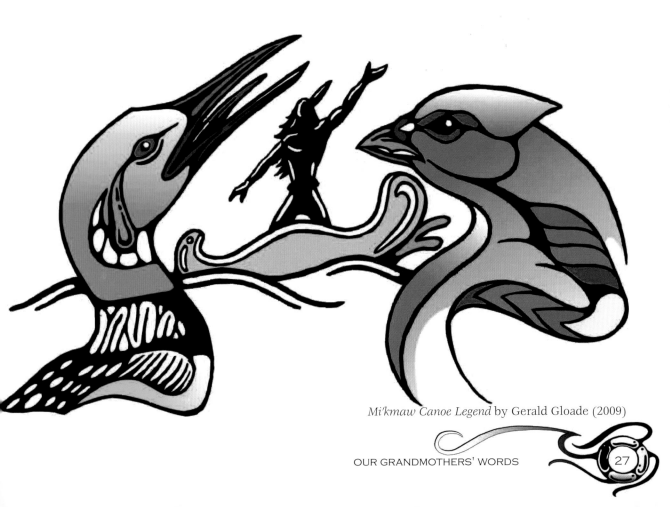

Mi'kmaw Canoe Legend by Gerald Gloade (2009)

Wkekkunitl telimtl, "Kikmanaq na maliamultaq. Kaqi-pilua'sitew ta'n teleyaskik. Kepmite'lmut na e'pit ta'n eskmalatl mijua'ji'jl. We'kaw wenik ta'n mu kesalulu'k wla'multaq nike' mita sespete'lma'titl mijua'ji'jl pema'lit. Aqq elmiaq ula mijua'ji'j weskwijinuij, kikmanaq apoqnmultaq nikwent."

Sali'j is sitting with her Godmother. Her Godmother reassures her, "The whole community will take care of you now. The attitude of everyone will change. It is a special thing when a woman is carrying a baby, a new life. Even people that sometimes aren't very nice to you – they will be nice to you now. They care about this baby as well. And when this baby is born, nurturing it is the responsibility of the whole community."

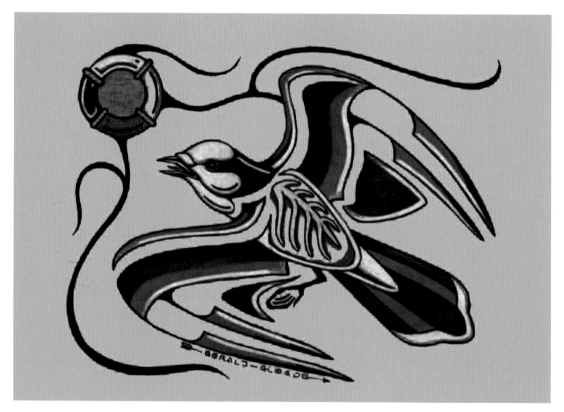

Kanata Jay by Gerald Gloade (undated)

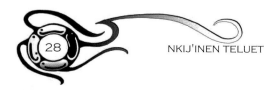

KA'QAWE'JI'J

Na to'q wikultisnik ka'qawejk. Te'si-eksitpu'k mawita'jik kulaman saqamaw kis-kinua'tuataq ta'n tett naji-ktantaqatitaq kiskuk. Kulaman ma' kaqianuk tami mijipjewey, te's na'kwek saqamaw elkimajik se'k nat-tuklultinew. Na te'si-eksitpu'k semaqkimujik nat-tuklultinew aqq elmi-wela'kw msit mawita'jik mawatalultinew.

Newte'jk eksitpu'k ka'qawe'ji'j elietl saqamawl telimatl, "Etuk kisi- naji-ktantekek elt ni'n? Telte'tm tepipunai kisi-ktanteken." Na saqamaw telimatl, "A' naji-ktanteke. Nattuklitesk." Mita saqamaw mu ketu'-l'kimaqal knekk, elkimatl wejuowk etek sitmuk. Saqamaw ekinua'tuatl, "Ta'n tujiw ika'n pemamkiaq we'jittesk kaqi-tepiaq milamu'k nme'juey. Pikwelkik nme'jk, e'sik aqq mn'tmu'k eymu'tijik na'te'l aqq elmiaq tepiejik ne'pe'j jukwa'latesk malqumanew wlo'nuk.

Welte'lsit ka'qawe'ji'j, klapis elt nekm ktantekewinu. Eliet pemamkiaq, welqatk ti. We'jiajik pikwelkik e'sik aqq ke'sk pem-mawo'laj wjit wikmaq nespiw pikwelkik kespa'lajik. Tepnmaj, elma'lajik weskwiejik wjit wikmaq wloqatalultinew.

Piluey eksitpu'k ika'q wije'wajik ktantekewinu'k naji-ankama'titl saqamawl kulaman kis-tlimaten ta'n tett kiskuk l'kimaten naji-ktantaqatinew. Ta'n tujiw saqmaw ekinua'tuaj ta'n tett lielital kiskuk, ka'qawe'ji'j tela'sit staqa

THE STORY OF CROW

There is a village of crows. Every morning the hunters gather and the Chief directs where they are to hunt today. To ensure there is always enough food, the Chief makes sure that the hunters don't go back to the same hunting ground they were on yesterday, or where any of their brothers had recently been. So each morning the hunters are dispersed to hunt and bring home food, and every evening the whole village gathers around to join in a feast.

One morning a young Crow approaches the Chief and says, "I want to go hunting too. I am of age now." So the Chief says, "Alright, you can hunt. You can bring us some food," but he doesn't want to send him very far, so he sends him to the sandbar. The Chief tells him, "When you get to the sandbar you will find fish or clams or oysters … any seafood, and when you have enough to bring home then come home and we will all have enough food to eat tonight."

The Crow is so excited – to be a hunter at last! He goes to the sandbar and feels great. He finds a lot of clams and while he is gathering them for the village he also eats a lot of them. When he is full, he brings the rest back to the village to be part of the evening feast.

The next morning he gathers with the other hunters before the Chief to be dispersed to the hunting ground for that day. But when Crow learns where to go, he nods his head and then ignores what the Chief has told him. He doesn't welte'teket na'sɨk ki's kisita'sit elistuan saqamawl. Mu eliek ta'n elkimuj, awnaqa apaja'sit pemamkiaq.

Tewji-wiklkik e'sɨk amujpa apaja'sit tlia'j na se'k elkimup. Na newtikiskɨk malqumajik e'sɨk. Ta'n tujiw awsamatalk, pe' atlasmit tujiw ki's app ketaqama'sit. Ta'n tujiw elmiet, mu koqoey aptuklik. Ka'qawejk na kesatmi'tij al-ke'kupio'lti'tij tami, nmiatesk al-ke'kupio'ltijik pemtaqtekl qasawo'qapi'l kisna psetkunn na'sɨk awisiw newtuka'lukutijik, kesatmi'tij mawkopia'ti'tij. Ki's piskiaq wela'kw ka'qawe'ji'j elmiet, mu koqoey pekisituk. Na elayja'sit psetkunn aqq newtukopit. Wkwijl wikumjl, "Juku'e kwi's amujpa mijisin, ma' na'te'l kispmkopiwun iapjiw!" Na'sɨk mu matpik ka'qawe'ji'j.

Ki's app piluey na'kwek ika'q, ka'qawe'ji'j ketu' apaja'sit pemamkiaq. Telta'sit kisi-kiseywatalq saqmawl, wkwijl aqq msɨt wikmaq. Na kesi-eksitpu'k semaqa'sit. Ta'n tujiw ktikik ka'qawejk mawita'tij kinua'tuksinew ta'n naji-ktantaqatitaq mu eymuk ka'qawe'ji'j. Saqamaw elietl ka'qawe'ji'jl wkwijl pipanimatl ta'n eymlij wkwisl. Teluetl, "Mu kejitu, semaqa'sipnaq atel wejkwapnia'q."

Elmi-wela'kw mu pekisinuk ka'qawe'ji'j. Msɨt wen sespite'lmatl aqq wkwijl sikteta'sitl. Msɨt tami alayja'sit telimajik wenik, "Mna'q nkwis pekisinuk, Mna'q nkwis pekisinuk." Klapis piskiaq, aqq mɨta ka'qawejk mu alayjita'qik tepkik, kejitutij ma' na nuku' pkisinukl

go where he is supposed to go – he goes back to that same sandbar.

He loved those clams so much he wanted to go back, even though he had been sent elsewhere. And all day he eats. He fills himself up, then he rests and eats again. When he goes back to the village, he is empty handed. He has nothing. Now, crows, they like to perch. You will often see them on wires or boughs, and they are hardly ever alone. They like to sit there with other crows. But that night, when the young Crow comes home late and brings no food, he flies up and sits on a bough all alone. He is not hospitable and he will not join the group – he just sits there on his perch alone, falling asleep. His mother calls him, "Come on down, you have to eat. You can't sit there forever!" But the Crow just sits there.

The next day, Crow wants to go back to the sandbar again. He thinks that he can fool the Chief, and his mother, and all of the village, so, very early, he flies away. When the other hunters gather to be dispersed to the hunting ground of the day, Crow was not there. The Chief goes to the old lady. "Where is your son?" he asks. She tells him that her son took off early, before dawn.

That evening, the Crow does not come back to the village. Everyone is concerned and the old lady is terrified. She flies around saying, "My son has not come home, my son has not come home." Finally it is dark and as Crows do not usually fly at night all of the village

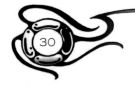
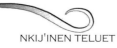

elmitpa'q. "Saqamaw telimajik, "Jenita'q. Eksitpu'nuk ni'n naji-kwiluates."

Eksitpu'k, ne'wt kaqi-pqutkimaj ktantekewinu'k, Saqamaw telimatl kisikui'skwl, "Keji'k ta'n eyk ɨkwis." Na saqamaw poqtamka'sit eliet pemamkiaq. Ta'n tujiw ika't pemamkiaq nemiajik e'sɨk ketmaqsetasijik alamkɨpultijik. Pikwelkl pitlanji'jl kis-mawamko'ttasikl we'jitoql, ka'qawe'ji'j kespa'lasni'k e'siki'k. Saqamaw pemukwatk pemapaqpilijik e'sɨk mi'soqo ika'j etl-kaqiaq pemamkiaq, na we'jiataq ka'qawe'ji'jaq. Neplisnaq. Ke'sk oqomita'sij aqq elistuaj saqamawl aqq setamk ika'laj wikmaq, nepkaq.

Ka'qawejo'q pane'smatek
Pemamkiaq eliesnaq
Naji-ankamujel nepkisnaq.

knows that he will not be arriving home. The Chief tells everyone, "Calm down. I will look for him in the morning."

So in the morning, after he has given his orders, the Chief tells the old lady, "I know where he is," and he leaves the village and goes to the sandbar. When he gets to the sandbar he sees mounds of clam shells everywhere. They are on both sides of the sandbar, big piles that the young Crow ate. The Chief follows the mounds of shells and at the very end of the sandbar, next to some empty clam shells he finds the Crow, dead. Ignoring the Chief's orders, ignoring the need of the village, he ate all the clams himself and died from greed.

When crow went digging for clams
He went to the shore
When they went to see him he had died.

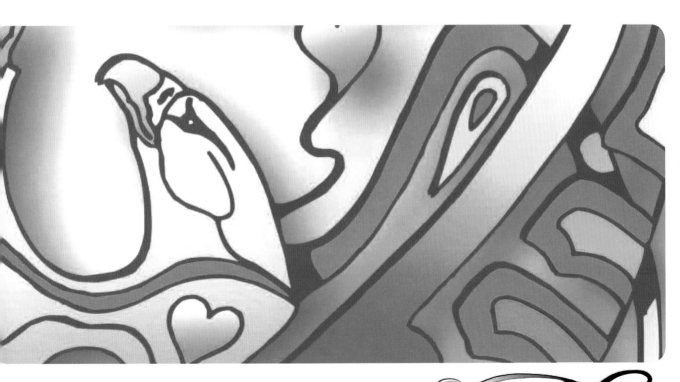

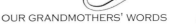

WILL I GET LOST?

Throughout the pregnancy, they all warn her, "Do not stand in a doorway or stand too long at a window when you are pregnant. You will develop an energy of stagnation that will not be kind when the baby is coming into the world. Your baby may get stuck and take a long time to be born. For the sake of you and your baby do not stand in a doorway or too long at a window." They tell her the stories that she remembers hearing as a child and she laughs when they remind her of how she learned to put her shoes on the correct feet.

Her Grandmother reminds her that the Mi'kmaw way of teaching is very subtle. "When you were little and learning how to put your shoes on the right foot, you would sit down, put them on, and then stand up, but before they left the house you would turn to me and say, 'Kiju. Am I going to get lost?'"

"And I would look at your feet and if the shoes were on the wrong feet I'd say, 'Yes.'"

"That was all I had to say and you would sit back down, and switch your shoes around to the other foot."

"And when the shoes were on the right feet then when you asked if you would get lost, I'd say, 'No, you are alright, you won't get lost.' And then you would happily leave the house. There is no harsh way of teaching how to put on your shoes, and you never tell a child that they are wrong. We Mi'kmaq have very subtle ways of teaching that every action always has a consequence that will affect you as well as others."

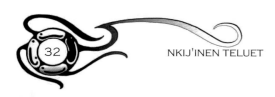

NKIJ'INEN TELUET

ETUK KSIKA'TES?

Teli-pkiji-skmaqtmaj msit wen telimatl, "Mukk taqmoqpukuiw ka'qnek kisna tewatpo'jinu tuopiti-iktuk ta'n tujiw eskmaqtman. Jiptuk elmiaq we'jitan mijua'ji'j taqmoqa'sitew kisna aptitesintew tujiw kitnmatesk tel-we'jitan." Na kisi-pkwatu'n mukk taqmoqpukuiw ka'qnek kisna tewatpo'jinu tuopiti-iktuk kulaman ki'l aqq knijan wle'toqsip.

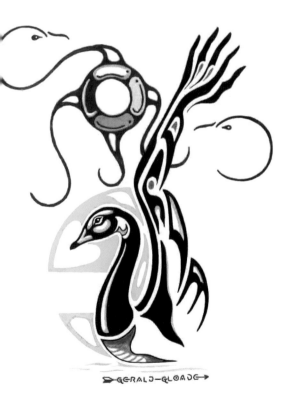

L'nu'k na mu nepuko'lti'k ta'n tel-kina'mua'tij. Apje'jit mijua'ji'j ekina'masit tetpaq-nasa'lan wmuksnk, pmkopa'sitew aqq nasa'lataq wmuksnk tujiw qama'sitew aqq ke'sk mna'q siaw-tu'ek kiwasklapa'sitew aqq pipanikesitew, "Kiju' ksika'tes?"

Ankaptmatl wkwatl aqq elmikjinaskuaj wmuksnk na telimt, "E'e."

Na na'msit amujpa telimt, na apatkopa'sitew aqq ilnasa'lataq wmuksnk.

Aqq tetpaqnaskuaj wmuksnk ta'n tujiw pipanikesit etuk ksika'tew, na pasik telimt, "Moqo, ma' ksika'win." Na siaw- tu'etew. Mu meta'luewun ta'n tel-kina'mat mijua'ji'j tetpaqnasa'lan wmuksnk, aqq mu telimawt mu tetpaqa'q. Mu nepukwe'nuk ta'n tel-kina'muemk ta'n wen tela'teket. Keknue'k wije'ti'tij ta'n tlitpietew nekm kisna wen piluey.

Kanata Goose by Gerald Gloade (undated)

 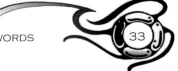

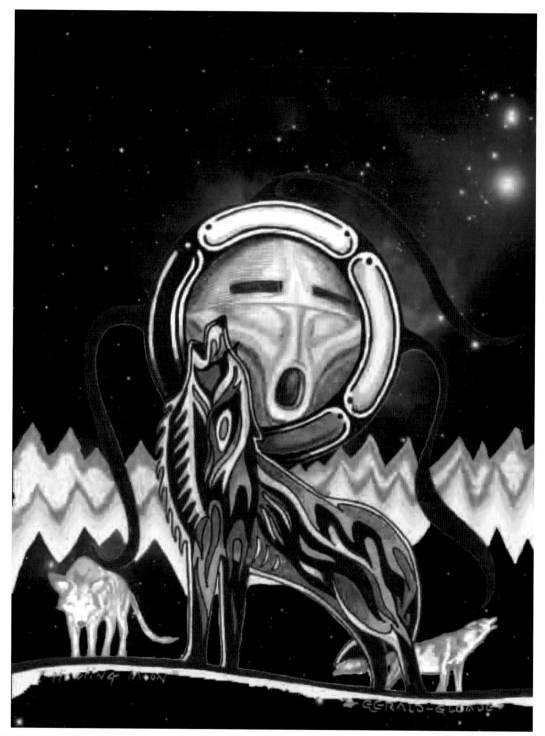

Margaret's Dogs by Gerald Gloade (undated)

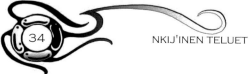

JI'NM TA'N EYK TEPKNUSET-IKTUK

Elapa'sij wen tetaqasitl tepknusetl, nmitatl ji'nml. Ula ji'nm na l'nu aqq nike' aknutmultes ta'n tel-kis-ika'j tepknuset-iktuk.

Na' to'q ula e'pit we'jitasnl l'pa'tujl. Na ula e'pit kesalatl wkwisl aqq kaqi-wineywatl. Klapis l'pa'tuj metu'qamiksit. Na wskwijinu'k aqq kisiku'k telima'titl e'pitl, "Amujpa na ekina'mat na kkwis." E'pit telimajik, "Ma' kis-tla'tekew na, awsami ksalk mta'lan. Awsami ksite'limk paqiatkoman ta'n tujiw o'pla'tekej."

Na l'pa'tuj metu'qamiksit. Wekayik aqq se'skwet aqq poqnitpaqa'lsit mu mesnmuk ta'n koqoey menuekej. Aqq wkwijl iknmaj ta'n pasɨk koqoey menuekelij. Menuekej koqoey ankmayiw e'pit weji-msnmuaj. Klapis tetuji winqamiksitl kisa'latl wkwisl, jel mu nuku' kejituk ta'n koqoey menuekej. Msɨt koqoey menueket!

Pemikwet pemi-aji-pepsite'lmatl wkwijl. Jijuaqa na almimatl kisna ewilwi'tatl wkwijl. E'pit meskimtl wkwisl na'sɨk telimsit, "Tetuji-ksalk ula l'pa'tuj mu ketu' mta'laq. Mu menuekew wkwayin kisna ewlita'sin. Awsami-ksite'lmk taliman."

Na mu talimaql, asite'lmatl tla'tekelin ta'n tel-mnuekelij.

Na'sɨk kisiku'k telima'titl, "Amujpa na ilumt mɨta mu kina'muawj winqamiksitew kisikwej."

THE MAN IN THE MOON

Many people look up at the full moon and see a man, and it is actually a Native man and now I'll tell you how he got there.

This is a legend of our people. There is a young boy and when he is born his mother just loves him so much, she spoils him rotten. He is a very spoilt child and the people tell her and the Elders tell her, "You have to discipline your son," but she says, "No, no, no, I love him too much to discipline him. I love him too much to tell him he is wrong when he does things."

So the boy often acts up and he screams and he hollers and he throws tantrums if he doesn't get his way. And his mother always gives him everything that he wants. If he wants something then she just does it for him right away without even asking. And she spoils him so bad that he doesn't even know what he wants ... he just wants everything!

As he grows, he becomes very disrespectful toward her. Sometimes he swears at his mother or calls her names. She is upset but she says, "I love him so much that I don't want him to be upset, I love him so much that I don't want him to get mad and I don't want to tell him off. I love him so much."

So she lets him be.

But the Elders tell her, "You have to discipline him because if you don't discipline him he is going to grow up to be a very mean man."

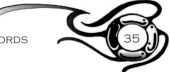

Aqq kisikwejek, ketloqo winqamiksit. Maqe'k aqq kesatk matnaket. Almimajik wenik aqq maqeywajik. Maqe'kɨp mijua'ji'juijek. Nike' ali-ksmekejik mijua'ji'jk ta'n tetpo'lti'tijik. L'pa maqe'k.

Na newte'jkek na'kwek eliet wkwijl wikilij. Kaquiet aqq poqji-paqiatkomatl wkwijl. E'pit telita'sit, "Mu ketu'-wkwaya'laq, awsami ksite'lɨmk." Na'sɨk poqji-se'skwalatl wkwijl aqq kesmeketl. Ta'n tujiw ma'minu keskmekej na nisielitl aqq wunji ika'q kun'tal etekl nu'te'lmaqn-iktuk. Na e'pit elisink l'pa mu aja'sik. Na ji'nm kwetayatl. Wetnu'kwalsit kis-tukwa'lan, na'sɨk me'si-tukwa'latl. Poqji-se'skwalatl, "Kiju', Kiju', mnja'si." Na'sɨk mu menja'silikl mɨta neplitl. Na kejitoq ne'pa'taq ke'sk wekayik. Mu weji-tla'tekekɨp na'sɨk tewji-wkwayikɨp kesmekepn ma'minu. Mu kejituk ta'n tla'teketew. Klapis kejitoq na tujiw pekisulj tel-lue'wit.

Na we'kwata'sit, wesimkwat aqq najikasit kisoqe'k. Aqq ke'sk etlikasit me'si puni-ankite'tk ta'n kis-tla'tekej aqq meskita'sit. "Mu nuta'nuksipnek tetuji-wkwayin. Tala'teketes nike'?" telita'sit.

Kisu'lkw kejiatl ta'n kis-tla'tekelij aqq meskeyatl, mɨta Kisu'lkw tel-

And when he gets older guess what happens? Exactly what the Elders said: he grows up to be a very mean man, and he always fights people and is just mean! He swears at people and he is a bully. He was a bully as a child too! He would push little kids, he would push people his own age. He is just mean.

Now, one day, when he is grown up, he goes into his mother's wikuom. He is in a bad mood and is saying mean things. She thinks, "Oh, I don't want him to be upset. I love him so much." But he starts hollering at her and he pushes her! And, when he pushes her, he pushes hard and she falls down and, when she falls down, she bangs her head. You know where the rocks are in the centre of the wikuom where the fire is? Well, when he pushes her she bangs her head on the rock. And now she just lies there and it scares him.

And he tries to wake her up but she won't wake up. He gets so angry and he tries waking her up and he says, "Mom, mom, get up! Mom, please get up!" but she can't get up. She can't get up because she is dead. He has killed her, with all of his anger. He didn't mean to but he was very angry and he pushed her. Now, he doesn't know what to do and he is thinking and he says, "Oh, my goodness. I don't know what to do now. My anger has done this."

And he gets very scared and he runs away to the woods. And while he is in the woods he keeps thinking about what he did and he feels bad and says, "I should never have been that angry. But now I don't know what to do."

Now Creator knows what has happened and he is really hurt by this

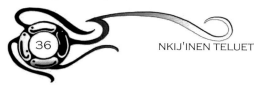

kina'muksi'k amujpa weleyajik knijink aqq weleyajik knki'kuk aqq mu puksiwkwayiwun. Kisu'lkw meskeyatl ula ji'nml ta'n kisi-tla'laj wkwijl. Na eliet kisoqe'k ta'n eymlij aqq pipanimatl, "Tallukwen ula tett?"

Ji'nm telimatl, "Etlikasi mita jipalul. Ne'pe'kaq nkijaq aqq meskeyi, na'sik mu kejitu ta'n tl-kinua'tultes tetuji-msikeyi."

Kisu'lkw telimatl, "Kejitu ta'n tl-kinua'tuitesk tetuji- msikeyin. Katu mikwite'te'n pkija'teketew. Etuk jel pitui-mtlnaqnipunqekl kisna newtiska'q te'sikl pitui-mtlnaqnipunqekl tli-pkije'ktitew na'sik kejitu ta'n tli-apiksitesk."

"Amujpa eltu'n nu'te'lmaqn aqq pekitnmatimkewey wasoqa'tu'n aqq tmaqn kwetmalt tujiw alasutman. Alasutmelsewt msit wen aqq alasutmelsewsin.

"Ma' kisi-asite'lmulu siawqatmn wsitqamu'k mita kisi-me'ki-o'pla'teken aqq ma' kisi-liewun wa'so'q mita me' mimajin. Etuk tala'lultes?"

Na kukumijinu tepknuset wejkwi-sekewa't kelusa'sit, "Kejitu ta'n tla'latesk ni'n. Wsua'lates naji-tkweywin. Tleywates staqa nuji'j aqq maliamates, tekweywitew aqq alasutmatew. Kisi wasoqa'tew pekitnmatimkewey aqq

man's actions because Creator believes that you should love your children, but you should also love your parents and should not be angry all the time. So he is really hurt about the man who pushed his mother. And goes into the dark woods, where the man is hiding in the dark woods. Creator asks him, "What are you doing?"

The man answers, "I am hiding because I am afraid of you. I killed my mother and I am sorry and I don't know how to say I am sorry."

And Creator says, "I have a way for you to say that you are sorry, but you have to remember it is going to take you a very, very long time. It may take you thousands of years. It may take you tens of thousands of years but I know how you can say I am sorry.

"You are going to have to light a fire and you are going to have to light a smudge and you are going to have to take a pipe and you are going to have to smoke it and you are going to have to pray. You are going to have to pray for all the people and you are going to have to pray for yourself.

"But I have a dilemma. I can't let you stay on the earth, but I can't take you to heaven because you are still alive, but I can't let you stay on the earth because what you did was so wrong. I wonder what I'll do?"

Now Grandmother Moon is just coming up on the horizon and she says, "I know what to do. I'll take him and he will stay with me. I'll be his Grandmother and I will look after him, and he can stay with me and he can pray. He can have his smudge bowl and

tmaqn aqq alasutmelsewsitew aqq alasutmelsewataq msit wenik."

Na nike' elapa'sin tetaqasit tepknuset, nmiatesk me' eyk na ji'nm etli-alasutmat iapjiw. I'tew na'te'l etli-aniapsit mi'soqo mu i'muk tepknuset aqq kaqiaq wsitqamu mita na Kisu'lkw telsutkis tla'sin.

can have his pipe and he can continue praying for himself and for the people."

So now, when we look at the full moon, we can see that he is there in the moon, praying for eternity. He will be there until there is no moon left and no earth left but he is there making his amends for that is where Creator put him forever. And if you look at the full moon that is where you will see him.

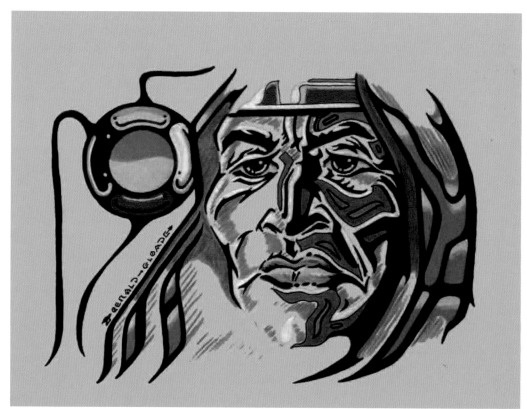

Kluskap by Gerald Gloade (2010)

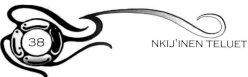

*K*iskuk pemkopia'tijik patawti-iktuk. Sali'j kewisink. Wi'kuama'titl mita telimajik naji-mesuktaqnat, l'pa mu tepnmaq. Aqq elp ketutamit. Telimajik, "L'pa tetuji-ktutmann wenju'su'nl mu sespete'tmu ta'n telamu'kl, stoqnamu'kl, mekwe'kl kisna tupkwanamu'kl, ketutman msit!" Wkekkunitl telimtl, "Elmiaq ketutamin, amujpa malqutmn ta'n koqoey ketutmn kisna knijan ala'tew klitam."

Keknue'k tetpaqatalumk Eskmalj Mijua'ji'j

*T*oday they are sitting around the dinner table. Sali'j is hungry. They are laughing because she says that she is hungry all the time lately. "I even have cravings for specific food. All this week I have wanted to eat apples. Big juicy apples. It doesn't matter if they are green, red, brown, I just want to eat them!" "You must satisfy a craving right away," her Godmother advises. "What you eat is important when you are pregnant."

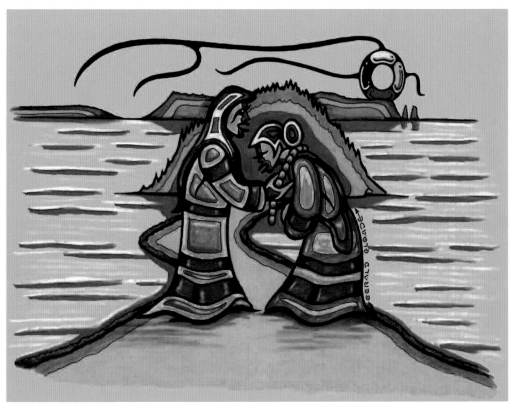

Partridge Island by Gerald Gloade (undated)

 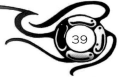

A'tukwaqn wjit Skusi'skwaq ta'n Malie'wi'tipnik Kloqoejk

Na' to'q wikijik. Te'si-wela'kw kesatmi'tij ankama'tij koqoejk. Na newte'jkek na'kwek ta'n tujiw ji'nmuk smaqita'tij naji-ktantaqatinew tapusijik e'pite'sk, ela'tijik kisoqe'k naqtmi'tij ta'n wikulti'tij.

Na pem-aknutmajik aqq weskewe'kik. Skusi'skwaq kesi-wape'kik staqa skus telamuksit kesik. Wijikitijik ula e'pite'sk. Ta'n tujiw poqji-piskiaq na aji-kisikuite'w Skusi'sk mimatua'toq ketkunimk aqq aji-nutqwe'te'w eltoq nu'te'lmaqn.

Kisi-poqnitpaqiaq, na Skusi'skwaq ankama'tijik kloqoejk aqq aknima'tijik. Aji-kisikuite'w Skusi'skw telimatl wkwe'ji'jl, "Kloqoejk na wskwijinu'k wikultijik maqamikew teluisik Kloqoeju'aq. Pasik nemitu'kl wpukwikual ankamuksi'kik." Na aknutmajik aqq eltu'titl a'tukwaqn wjit kloqoejk nemia'tijik.

Na aji-nutqwe'te'w Skusi'skw pipanimatl wmisl, "Teken ki'l welamt?" Na wmisl telimtl "Nemi't ala' mawi-ksasit kloqoej, nekm na Kitpu. Welapit aqq kelu'sit ktantekewinu. Nekm ni'n welamk aqq ajipjutm malie'winen." Nutqwe'te'w telimatl wmisl, "Mu nekm ni'n welamaq. Welamk ni'n ala' mekwasit kloqoej, nekm na Pipukwes." Na aknima'tijik kloqoejk mi'soqo klapis nepasni'k jel elistesinki'k Wjipenuk.

Ke'sk nepa'tij, Kitpu aqq Pipukwes peji-miskua'tijik wte'pitemuaq aqq elma'la'tijik ta'n wiki'tij Kloqoeju'aq.

THE STAR BRIDES

One morning, when the men have gone out to hunt, two women walk off deep into the forest and leave their camp.

They are happy, these two women. They are Skusískwaq, Weasel Women, and their skins are very white, like every Weasel Person's fur is in the wintertime. And these two Skusískwaq are sisters. Older Sister takes them deep into the forest, and there she builds a shelter-camp. Younger Sister makes a small fire.

Now it is night. The sun has gone beneath the earth, and those two Weasel Sisters are lying there looking up at the stars. Older Sister says to Younger Sister, "Those are people up in the Sky World. Look at their eyes, shining up there."

Younger Sister says, "Which one would you like to have for your husband? One with big eyes, or one with little eyes?"

Looking into the night sky, Older Sister says, "I choose that one there, the shiniest and brightest."

"Oh, that one!" Younger Sister says, "That one is ugly."

"So," says Older Sister. "So then. Which one would you have?"

"I will have that little star there, the little red one."

And then these two Weasel Women fall asleep, looking toward the east, where their two stars are hunting across the night.

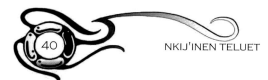

Eksitpu'k tukiet nutqwe'te'w skusi'skw. Na ta'n tujiw kiwaskisma'sij na'tuenl kelultl. Telimtl, "Anko'te'n tela'teken, suel kutateskat wijke'tlaqn ta'n etek npisun wjit npukwikl." Wenaqipsu'kwa't Skusi'skw, nemiatl mekwalkikwatl kisikuo'pji'jl epilitl. Nekm na Pipukwes, mekwasite'w kloqoej ta'n kisi-mknapn wela'kwek.

Ktik Skusi'skw elp tukiet. Na ta'n tujiw kiwto'qisma'sij na'tuenl kelultl. Telimtl, "Anko'te'n tela'teken, suel kutateskat wijke'tlaqn ta'n etek sekwan a'maqanm nsiskwek." Wenaqpsu'kwa't Skusi'skw nemiatl pitoqsitl ji'nml epilitl. Nekm na Kesasite'w kloqoej ta'n kisi-mknapn wela'kwek.

Na Skusi'skw tekweywa'tijik wji'numumuaq. Naji-kisikuite'w Skusi'skw telimatl wji'numuml, "Mu koqoey ala'tu wisku'pulnin." Telimtl, "Mu kewisinuek, ktaqama'titesnen api-ktantekeyek, nujo'tmuk puktew aqq maliaptmuk koqoey mi'soqo apaja'tiek. Katu mukk sama'tup kun'tew etek kikjuk wikuomk." "A', ma' tala'tuek aqq wissukwateketesnen," teluejik Skusi'skwaq.

Na telo'ltijik, te'sikiskik ji'nmuk semaqa'tijik naji-ktantekejik aqq

Now it is morning. Younger Sister stretches under her furs; she is waking up. Her foot touches something. "Be careful!" cries a little squeaking voice. "You have upset the bark dish of nepíjekwati, the medicine for my eyes." Younger Sister sits up. Who has spoken? By her side is a little old man, with a wrinkled face and sore red eyes. It is that small red Star Person. By talking in the night, she has called him to be her husband. She has called the Star With Sore Eyes.

Now Older Sister begins to wake up. She moves a little under her sleeping robes. "Watch out!" says a man's voice. It is a deep strong voice. "You have upset the bark dish with my sikwan, my red ochre." Older Sister rolls over and sits up. Lying there next to her is a tall, strong man. His face is painted with red ochre. It is her Star Husband, whom she has called to her by talking in the night. She has called the Star With Shining Eyes. So these two Weasel Women are to be the wives of Stars.

"I have nothing to give you to eat," says Older Sister. "We do not need to eat until we come home from hunting," says her husband. "You can gather wood and tend the fire, and prepare for our return. But there is one thing you must not do."

"Áa," says Younger Sister's Husband, the Star With Sore Eyes. "There is one thing you must not do. You must not move that flat rock which lies before the wigwam. You must not move it, you must not lift it."

"Very well," says Older Sister. "We will cook for you on your return."

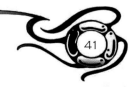

Skusi'skw nujo'tmi'tij puktew aqq
wissukewa'tijik wji'numumuaq.

Klapis poqji-siwqatkik. Mu tami
nemia'tikik wikmawaq. Newte'jkek
na'kwek ke'sk ali-ktana'tij sipeknk,
nutqwe'te'w Skusi'skw pipanimatl wmisl,
"Etuk koqoey etek lame'k na kun'tew?"

"Mukk tala'tu na kun'tew," telimtl
wmisl.

Na'sik mu punajutmuk nutqwe'te'w
Skusi'skw aqq klapis kisita'sit kimaptmn
ta'n koqoey etek lame'k na kun'tew.
Na eliet aqq aja'toq aqq pu'taptik.
"Koqoey nemitu'n?" pipanimtl wmisl.
Nutqwe'te'w Skusi'skw koqqwa'toq
wsiskw aqq poqji-se'skwet, "Tami eymu'k
nmis, tami apukwe eymu'k?"

Wmisl ejikliksma'litl aqq pu'taptmlij
ta'n kun'tew etekip. Na nemitoq
wsitqamu knekk pkewe'k etek, aqq
nemitoq kisitu'tip etli-ktuknimk ke'sk
mna'q elma'lukwi'tikek wji'numumuaq.
Na kejitoq eykik kloqoeju'aq. Kun'tew
apajiw ika'toq ta'n teltekip. Na
pe'skitemit Skusi'skw aqq wkwe'ji'jl
koqqwa'latl. Na kelnutijik aqq kitk
atkitemijik. Klapis mekwalqekl
wpukwikual tetuji-ma'muni-atkitemijik.

Knekk kisoqe'k wji'numumuaq
ketantekelijik. Kinapk na nekmowk. Na
ankmayiw kejitu'tij na'taliaq wikuaq.
Kejitu'tij wte'pitemuaq atkitemilijik.

Now many days go by. The Weasel
Women go out to look for sipeknk, the
ground-nuts, wild potatoes. They are
digging them up, they are going to cook
them. And Younger Sister is talking
again. "I wonder what is under that
stone?"

"You leave that flat stone alone," says
Older Sister.

But Younger Sister keeps talking
about it, and soon she has talked herself
right up to it, and soon she has talked
her hands right on it, and then she is
lifting it up.

She lifts the stone and looks under it.
"What is there?" asks Older Sister.
Younger Sister screams.
"Where are we?" shrieks Younger
Sister. "Where are we, my Older Sister?"

Older Sister pushes her aside, and
looks under the stone, looks to see what
is making her little Weasel Sister yell
so. And she sees: they are in the World
Above the Sky. They are standing on top
of the sky. The stone is covering a hole
in it, and through this hole she can see
down, down, down to the earth below,
to the forest, to the little shelter-camp
she built the night the two of them lay
talking together about the eyes of stars.

Older Sister bursts into tears.
Younger Sister bursts into tears. These
two Weasel Women weep until their eyes
are red with crying.

Way out in the forest of the World
Above the Sky, the Star Husbands
are hunting. And they begin to know
something, and feel that something is
wrong. They begin to feel their wives

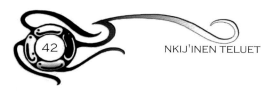

"Tepias apaji-l'ma'ti'k, aja'tu'tijek kun'tewek," telimtijik.

Pem-piskiaq pekisini'tij. Wte'pitemuaq tela'tijik staqa mu talianukek. Awnasi la'mua'tijik wji'numumuaq. Na'sik mu kiseywa'tikik. "Kis-na'taliaq kiskuk. Koqoey wjit atkitemioqsip?" pipanima'tijik Skusi'skwaq. Nutqwe'te'w Skusi'skw telimajik, "Mu talianuk. Mna'q atkitemiwek." Kitpu telimatl wte'piteml, "Amuj na'taliaq. Kisi-aja'tuoq kun'tew. Nemituo'q ta'n koqoey etek lame'k. Nike' ketu' l'ma'tioq." Mu kis-klusik Skusi'skw, ankamatl wji'numuml aqq waju'peka'tikl wpukwikl saqpikunn. Na telimtl, "Na to'q, apaji-l'makimultesnen."

Pipukwes telimaji, "Wlo'nuk naji-npayoq, anquna'toqsip kun'jewal. Eksitpu'nuk mukk jikleka'tup naqsunual aqq mukk panta'tup kpukwikual. Tmk nutuatoqsip Jijikes wetewintoq, mukk panta'tup kpukwikual. Tujiw nutuatoqsip Amalpaqme'j wetewintoq, mukk panta'tup kpukwikual. Pekije'k nutuatoqsip Atu'tuej wetewintoq, na tujiw kis-panta'tutoqsip kpukwikual."

crying. "We had better go back," says the Star Husband With Shining Eyes. "They must have lifted the stone," says the Star With Sore Eyes. "Listen to them crying."

It is almost evening when those Star Persons come out of the forest. Their Weasel Wives are trying to cook, trying to pretend that nothing has happened.

But Star Persons have power, and they know. "What has troubled you today?" they are asking their wives. What have you been crying about?"

"Nothing is wrong," says Younger Sister. "We have not been crying."

"Ah," says the husband of Older Sister. "I think you have been looking through the hole in the sky. I think you have been lifting the stone and looking down at your world. And I think that you are lonely and want to return to it."

Older Sister looks up at her Star Husband. She cannot say anything. She looks at him and tears start to come out of her eyes.

"Very well," he says to her. "You may go back to the earth world."

The old Star With Sore Eyes tells them, "Tonight you must sleep close together. You must keep your fur robes over your heads. And in the morning, when the sun comes from beneath the earth, you must lie very still. Do not take the robes from over your heads, do not open your eyes. First you will hear Jikiki the chickadee calling. Keep your eyes shut. Next you will hear Apalpaqmej, Red Squirrel Person, you will hear him singing. Do not open your eyes. After a long time, you will hear Atu'tuej, Striped Squirrel. He will sing, and then you may open your eyes."

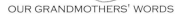 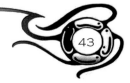

Kitpu teluet, "Tla'tekeyoq ta'n telkimulek apajiw i'toqsip wsitqamu'k."

Na Skusi'skwaq naji-npajik. Anquna'tu'titl wunjewal. Klapis eksitpu'k. Nutua'titl Jijikesl wetewintoql. Nutqwe'te'w Skusi'skw awnase'k ketu' menju'naqiet pasik wmisl petqa'matl. Pekije'k nutua'titl Amalpaqme'j wetewintulitl. Ki's app Nutqwe'te'w Skusi'skw ketu' menju'naqiet na'sik wmisl telimtl, "Pe' jenpi, amujpa eskmalu'k Atu'tuej mtewintun."

Klapis ki's app Amalpaqme'j wetewintoq. Nutqwe'te'w Skusi'skw telta'sit Atu'tuejl nutuatl na ejikleka'latl naqsunn aqq menju'naqiet. Na wetewse'skwetaq, "Tami eymu'k nmis?" Wmisl menjapietl, eykik apajiw wsitqamu'k na'sik awsami wisqi-mnja'titki'k, knekk kmu'j-iktuk ke'kupijik. Mu etenukl psetkunn ta'n tl-niskusua'titaq. Aptito'kwejik ke'kwe'k kmu'j-iktuk. Aqq ta'n tujiw nutaj wju'sn kmu'j-iktuk, mu na wju'sn nutmu'n, nutajik na Skusi'skwaq wesku'tmi'tij ta'n tl-nisa'titaq.

"If you do this," says the tall Star Husband, "you will find yourselves back in your shelter-camp, the place you were lying the night you invited us to come and be your husbands."

So these two Weasel Women lie and cover their heads with sleeping robes. The night passes, and in the morning they hear the chickadee. Younger Sister, always impatient, wants to leap up, but Older Sister forces her to lie still. "Wait! Wait until we hear Atu'tuej," she says.

After a long while they hear something singing. What is it? It is Apalpaqmej, Red Squirrel. And that foolish Younger Sister, she jumps at the noise and throws off the covers. "Where are we, my Older Sister?" Older Sister sighs and opens her eyes. The sun has come from beneath the earth, and these Weasel Women are back in their own world. But they have opened their eyes too soon on the way down, and now they are stuck in the top of a tall, tall pine tree, a kuow tree. There are no branches in this tree, except a few at the very top, and these two women cannot get down. And maybe when we hear the whispering in the tops of the pine trees, it is not the wind, but it is the two Weasel Women Sisters planning how they will find their way down the tree.

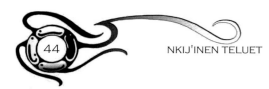

Siawa'lik, Nsi'sk, Siawa'lik!

Na' to'q, wikultisni'k kisikui'skw aqq ne'sijik wkwisk wikuom-iktuk. Aji-kisikuite'wk wkwisk seskwe'kik aqq weliaponmasijik aqq apoqntmi'tij wikuow aqq wutanmuew. Attikna'tijik. Ketantu'tij wilu'ow, naqana'pejik aqq kaqi- maliaptmi'tij msit koqoey wjit wkwijual.

Katu maw-nutqwe'te'wl wkwisl mu tal-lukwelikl, pasik alkopietl wikuaq. L'pa mu tali-wtapsunik, mu apoqnmasik aqq mu apoqntmuk koqoey wikuaq kisna wutank. Elita'sualatl wkwijl maliamkun.

Eksitpu'k kisikui'skw tukwa'latl, ekno'tlatl aqq kiskaja'tuaj wilu, jel me nukjaqte'muaj wilu. Msit koqoey elukwatmuaj. Ktikik wkwisk telimjik, "Kiju' elmiaq mpimn amujpa wije'wultew mita ma' ninen kis-tleywaqit staqa ki'l teleyat. Amujpa ekina'mat maliamsin." Na'sik kisikui'skw mu ekina'muaql maw-nutqwe'te'wl wkwisl. Jel pemi-aji-male'kl, klapis jel mu kisi-ksispa'lsik, kisikui'skw amujpa ela'tuaj samqwan ksispa'lan.

Aji-kisikuite'wk wkwisk wekayikik, "Awsamiaq na nuku'," teluejik, "Awsama'sit na jel Nkijinen amujpa piskwapilk samqwan ksispa'lan. Wikit na nekm elt tett na'sik mu tali-apoqntmuk koqoey. Pasik elisink kikjuk nu'te'lmaqn aqq nepat." Aqq teliaq ta'n telue'tij, pasik elisink kikjuk nu'te'lmaqn, jijuaqa na katu kewaskisma'sit apu'smn wpaqam tujiw apajinpat."

Drive on, boys!

There are three sons who live with their mother in a wikuom. The two eldest sons are hard working and are always doing things for themselves, for the household and for everybody else. They always work hard. They hunt for food, they bring in water for the family, and they look after each other and their mother.

But the youngest son never does anything, apart from mope around the house. He never does anything to help himself or be an active part of his family or community. He is totally dependent on his mother.

She wakes him, and puts his clothes out for him. She fixes his food, and even mashes it for him like she did when her boys were babies. She does everything for him. Her eldest boys would say to her, "Mom, when you die, he is going to go with you because we are not going to be able to take care of him like you do. You have to get him to help himself." But the old lady never tries to discipline her youngest son. In fact, it gets worse because there comes a day when he doesn't even bother to wash himself, and so the old lady fetches a pan of water for him to wash in.

This makes the older boys upset. "Now he has gone too far," they say. "He has gone too far. Our mother bringing him a pot of water for him to wash! He is part of our family but he never does anything to help. All he does is sit by the fire and sleep." And they are right. All he does is sit and lie by the fire, occasionally turning around to warm his back, and then he sleeps again.

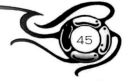

Klapis kisikui'sko'q nepkaq aqq wsisk telita'sijik wjiknamual elt npilital mita mu apoqnmasikl. Wenmajita'sit l'pa'tuj, l'pa mu tal-lukwek pasik atkitemuktuatl wkwijl. Ta'n tujiw pun-wenmajita'sit, me' mu tal-lukwek pasik elisink kikjuk nu'te'lmaqn, mu ketaqma'sik aqq mu kesispa'lsik. Mu menja'sik ksispa'lsin, klapis poqji-kslet. Wsisk klapis puni-wksayajik apoqnmasin kisna apoqntmn koqoey. Telimtijik, "L'pa mu tali-wtapsunik, mu apoqnmasik aqq mu apoqntmuk ta'n telo'ti'k. Pasik ne'likawet aqq keslema'toq ta'n wiki'k." Aqq teliaq na.

Na newte'jkek na'kwek ta'n tujiw elma'ti'tij wsisk, tetuji-kslek eymilij jel mu kaqmutmi'tik. Tewa'tu'titl wilu'al natatalkik kuwijmuk. "Tala'latesnu?" pipanimtijik. Ankite'tmi'tij ta'n tla'lataq wjiknamual, klapis kisa'matijik naji-pqwasekenew apaqtuk.

Na pija'la'titl mun'ti-iktuk wjiknamual, sepusepilmi'tij mun'ti aqq tepeke'tij setamk tapaqn-iktuk tujiw poqtamka'la'titl wjiknamual naji-pqwaseke'titl apaqtuk. Mu awsma kejitu'tik ta'n etek apaqt, na'sik ami-kjijitu'tij ta'n la'titaq. Knekk ika'jik mu wenl l'pa welteskua'tikl, klapis welteskua'titl nuji-ika'taquetl awtik.

Welta'suala'titl tujiw pipanima'titl, "Tali-amasek etek sitmuk aqq tali-ika'tesnen na'te'l?" Na kisikuo'p telimajik ta'n tl-teskitaq sitmuk aqq telimaji ma'

One day the old lady dies and the older boys reassure themselves that their younger brother is going to die too because he still does nothing to help himself. At first, he mourns for his mother and doesn't do anything else. And then when he finishes mourning for his mother he just continues to lie by the fire, not eating, not washing. He won't even get up to take a bath and after a few weeks he smells really bad! His brothers give up trying to encourage him to help himself or help them with the chores. They say, "He is no good to himself, no good to his family, no good to the community. He is just useless. All he does is occupy space and smell up the house." And it is true.

One day the older brothers come home and as they open the door to the wikuom they are hit with a smell that is so bad that they can't even stay in their home. They get their food and eat it outside. "What are we going to do?" they say. They think for a while and then they say, "We are going to throw him away. Let's take him to the ocean and throw him in the water."

So they put him in a burlap bag, tie it up, throw it in the back of their truck wagon and start their journey to the ocean. They are not exactly sure how to get to the ocean, but they know the direction they need to go in. They travel a long distance without seeing anyone else, and after several hours they meet a farmer beside the road.

After greeting him, they ask, "Can you tell us how far the shore is from here and how to get there?" So the old man is telling them the way and saying that

ika'qik tel-knekk kiskuk amujpa skmataq mi'soqo sapo'nuk. Na kisiku mikuaptik mun'ti i'-aja'sik.

Ki's app ankaptik aqq pipanimajik, "Wen pisit mun'tektuk?"

Telima'titl, "Njiknaminen na."

"Kjiknamuew? Tala'teket?"

"Ela'likit sitmuk naji-pqwasekeyek apaqtuk," telima'titl.

Pa'qalayik ti nuji-ika'taqut, pipanimajik "Koqoey wjit naji-pqwasekeyoq kjiknamuew?"

Telima'titl, "Mu eta l'pa tali-wtapsunik. L'pa mu koqoey kisa'tuk jel mu kisi-ktuapsik aqq mu wenl pilue'l kis-apoqnmuaql na naji-pqwasekeyak kulaman kaqi-lukwaqnitew."

Nuji-ika'taqut teluet, "Niskam, mukk jiklekip mimajuinu!"

Na'sik l'pa'tuj wsisk teluejik, "Amujpa tela'tekeyek. Me'jpa na npitew mita l'pa mu kisi-ktuapsik. Je mu kis-smsik."

Nuji-ika'taqut telimajik, "Tala'tekeyoq apuke. Mu na ejiklekewun mimajuinu. Ni'n ksua'lates aqq l'ma'lates."

"Ta'n tujiw mijisi elt nekm mijisitew. Kisi-apoqnmasij na pipnaqn tlawsitew."

Na mun'ti ki's app aja'sik aqq l'pa'tuj kelusa'sit, pipanimatl Nuji-ika'taqutl, "Kisjaqasik tipu'lewey aqq amjaqikn pipnaqn-iktuk?"

Nuji-ika'taqut telimatl, "Mu telte'tmu. Menueken tipu'lewey aqq amjaqikn amujpa ki'l eljaqmn pipnaqn-iktuk."

Na l'patuj wetew-pe'sklamit mun'tektuk tujiw teluet, "Siawa'lik, Nsi'sk, Siawa'lik!"

they probably won't make it to the ocean today – "maybe tomorrow morning" – when the burlap bag moves a little.

The farmer looks at it and says, "What do you have in the bag?"

"Oh, that is our brother," the boys say.

"Your brother? What is wrong with him?"

"We are taking him to the shore and throwing him in," they reply.

The farmer is shocked. "Now why would you do that?"

"Well," they say, "he is not able to help himself. He is not able to do anything for himself or for anyone else either, so we are going to throw him in the water."

And the farmer says, "Oh my goodness, don't throw a person away!"

But the boys say, "We have to. He is going to die anyway because he doesn't do anything for himself. He doesn't eat."

"What is the matter with you guys? You can't throw a person away. I will take him. I'll take him to my farm," says the farmer.

"When I eat, he'll eat too. If he can help himself to bread then he will live."

When he says this, the sack moves and a voice comes up out of it. "Will the bread have butter and jam on it?" says the voice.

The farmer says, "I don't think so. If you want to have butter and jam on it you must do it yourself."

There is a little sigh and from the sack the voice says, "Drive on boys, drive on."

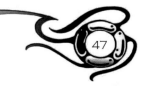

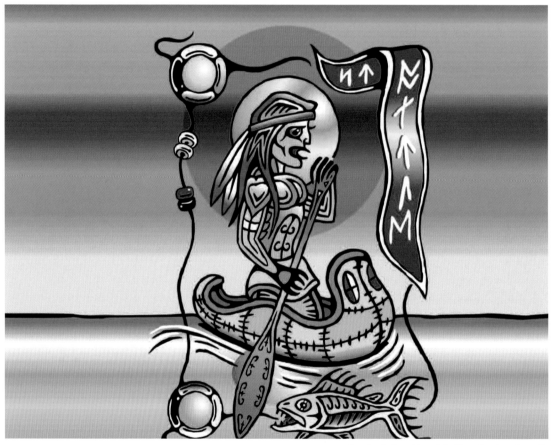

St. Antle by Gerald Gloade (undated)

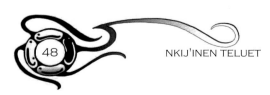

Ke'sk pemikwetl wunijan wmustek, Sali'j poqji-wskumatl. Kejitoq na' Mi'kmaq telo'ltijik.

Wkwijl telimtl, "Mi'kmaq na ne'kaw weskuma'titl mijua'ji'jl ke'sk mna'q weskwijinuilik. Weskumt, ekina'mat wjit ta'n telo'lti'k aqq wjit wsitqamu. Elmiaq pmkopa'sin pite'man kisna atlasmin, teluen 'Nijan pemkopa'ti'k aqq atlasmi'k kijka'. Keknue'k na atlasmimk aqq keknue'k ekinua'tat knijan ta'n tel-lukwen. Weji-nmitoq wsitqamu ki'l kpukwik aqq ne'kaw weskumt, ilajuktat wjit ta'n tujiw weskwijinuij. Mi'kmaq ketlamsitasultijik ta'n tujiw eskmaqtman mu kaqi-kinua'tuawt msit wen ta'n tel-militpien. Eyk koqoey pasik ki'l aqq knijan kejituoq. Mu al-ne'a'tu'n kmusti msit wen nmitun mita kepme'k eskmaqtmamk. Atel poqji-kitman kikmaq pasik ekinua'tajik eskmaqtman."

Sali'j teluet, "Teliaq teluen, atel poqti-kitmayanek pasik nikmaq ekinua'taqitipnik. Telo'tmas welta'suaqn ika'q ntinink, tujiw me' kne'kek ekinua'taqitipnik pilue'k wenik. Na tujiw wenik wutank welta'sultipnik ketu' wunijaniek."

Wkiju'eml weskewe'kl, "Pasik skma, elmiaq knijan weskwijinuij na tujiw nmittesk welta'suaqn. Kinu na Mi'kmaq nata'-wi'kipaltulti'k."

Ta'n Telqamiksin aqq Ta'n Tela'teken We'tua'lij Knijan.

As Sali'j grows bigger with her pregnancy she finds herself talking to the baby that she is carrying inside her body. She knows this is the Mi'kmaw way.

Her Mother told her, "We Mi'maq are talking to the baby all the time, before it is born. We talk to it and tell it all about things in our life and in our world. When you sit down for a break or a drink, you say, 'Well baby, we are going to sit and rest for a bit.' It is important to rest and important to tell the baby what is going on. You are its eyes, and all the time when you are talking you are preparing it for being born. You see, in our culture, pregnancy is very private. It is between the mother and the baby. It is not okay to be showing your belly off to everyone. It is an internal time, a deep time. During the first trimester only the family knows of the pregnancy."

"That is right," says Sali'j, "we only told a few people in our family for those first three months. It felt like there was a quiet celebration going on inside me all that time, and after the first three months then it became more of a community celebration that there is going to be a baby."

"Well, wait until that little baby is born," laughs her Grandmother, "then you will really know what it feels like to be part of that celebration. We Mi'kmaq know how to celebrate!"

How you act and what you do affects the baby.

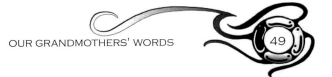

Lo'li Pusali

Ula a'tukwaqn wjit ta'n telitpiaqsɨp ki's sa'q Ktaqamkuk. Ktaqamkuk wutanji'j wikisnaq newtukwe'kaq l'pa'tu'saq. Mu witapik aqq mu weltesinuk tami. Katu mu kesi-sespɨte'tmuk, welqatk aqq mil-lukwet na'sɨk ksats witapij. Kaqi'sk eliet sitmuk aji-amalapit aqq almila'sit. Na ula na'kwe'k amalo'toql kun'tal apaqtuk na nutuatl na'tuenl elkomiktatl, "Lo'li Pusali! Lo'li Pusali! Ke' tl-wla'li apaji-pqwasa'li." Telsɨtuatl e'pitl wetewi-l'nui'sitl.

Lo'li nutuatl na'sɨk mu nemiaql wenl kikjuk na telta'sit telistaqnewa'sit na siawa'sit sitmuk. Mu knekk ika'q ki's app nutuatl na'tuenl elkomiktatl, "Lo'li Pusali! Lo'li Pusali! Ke' tl-wla'li apaji-pqwasa'li."

Loli Pusali

This is a story that happened in Newfoundland a long time ago. In a community in Newfoundland there is a young man who is always alone. He is a bit of an outcast and hasn't got any good friends. He is okay though and mostly happy, keeping busy, but he wishes he had more friends. Often he goes down to the shore, to walk and kick around in the sand. This day he is skipping rocks on the water when he hears something. "Loli Pusali! Loli Pusali! Please put me back in the water." It is a woman's voice and she is speaking Mi'kmaw.

Loli hears the words, but he can't see anyone close to him and he thinks he is imaging it, so he keeps on walking on the beach. But he only goes a few steps when he hears the voice again: "Loli Pusali! Loli Pusali! Please put me back in the water."

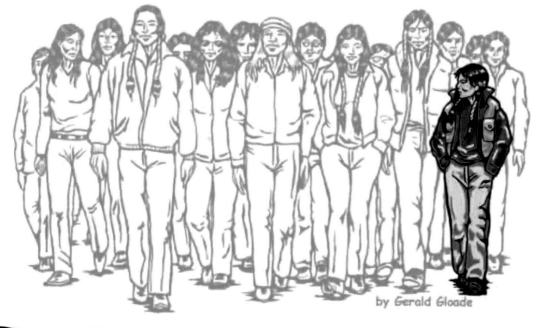

by Gerald Gloade

All My Relations by Gerald Gloade (undated)

Nike' poqji-awnasita'sit Lo'li. Etuk jel ketu'-kiseyajik mijua'ji'jk. Ki's app alapetesink na nemitoq na't-koqoey piltuamu'k sitmuke'l. Ta'n tujiw ika'j kikjuk nemiatl kelu'sitl Nme'juinu'skwal. Ke'kupiji tmoqta'wk elakweliji, aptito'kwet, me'si apaja'sit apaqtuk. Nemi'jl aqq elkomiktatl.

"Lo'li Pusali! Lo'li Pusali! Ke' tl-wla'li apaji-pqwasa'li. Npites aji-pkitqatman na'ku'setew-iktuk, ke' tl-wla'li apaji-pqwasa'li."

Lo'li eliet ta'n eymlij aqq nemitoq awsami-knekk qasqe'k eymilitl. "Telita'sit, Kis-tala'teketes ni'n? Tal-kisi-apoqnmuates ta ni'n? Mu ni'n wen."

"Ma' pkwanulnu," telimatl "aqq ma' pkwanaqik tmoqta'wk. Ejela'lul, ma' kisi-apoqnmulu." Na Lo'li ejiklika't. Mu knekk ika'q ki's app nutuatl elkomiktatl, "Lo'li Pusali! Lo'li Pusali! Ke' tl-wla'li apaji-pqwasa'li."

"Ki's telimulap, ejela'lul, ma' kisi-apoqnmulu." Na si'stewey Lo'li ejiklika't na'sik me elkomiktatl. "Lo'li Pusali! Lo'li Pusali! Ke' tl-wla'li apaji-pqwasa'li."

Na telita'sit, "Ma' jiksituaq," aqq siawa'sit na'sik pemi-aji-ksikawisawetl mi'soqo klapis telimsit, "A', apaja'sites aqq ankaptites ta'n kis-tla'teketes."

Na Lo'li apaja'sit ta'n ula Nme'juinu'skw ke'kupilij tmoqta'wk. Pipanimatl, "Tal-kisi-pkwanultes? Mu ni'n melkiknaw, ni'n na menaqnay aqq mu wenewiw."

Na'sik poqji-kwetnajik tmoqta'wk, aqq pekije'k mu tmoqta'wk ajita'qik. Kaqi-ika'lsit Lo'li kwetnasit na jijuaqa tmoqta'wki'k ajita'tki'k, elmi

Now Loli is really confused. Maybe it is some kids playing a trick on him. He looks around and notices that there is something strange over there on the sand. He goes closer and sees it is a beautiful mermaid. She is sitting on a pile of logs, stranded away from the water. She has seen him and he hears her calling to him. "Loli Pusali! Loli Pulasi! Please put me back in the water. I'll die if I sit in this sun. Please put me back in the water."

Lo'li goes up to her and sees that she is far from the water. He thinks, "What can I do? How can I help her? I'm a nobody, I'm nothing."

"I can't even lift you up," he tells her. "I can't lift those logs. I can't do anything, I can't help you," and he starts walking away. But again he hears her "Loli Pusali! Loli Pulasi! Please put me back in the water."

"I told you," he says, "I told you I can't help you." And he starts walking away a third time when he hears, "Loli Pusali! Loli Pulasi! Please put me back in the water."

So he says to himself, "I'm going to ignore her," and he keeps walking away, but she calls louder and louder, until finally he says to himself, okay, I'll go back and see what I can do.

So Loli goes back to the mermaid sitting on the logs, and he says to her, "How can I lift you? I'm not strong, I'm a weakling, I'm a nobody."

But Loli starts tugging at the logs anyway, and for a long time it seems that nothing is going to budge them or move them. He is tugging at the logs,

nisoqomkietki'k samqwan-iktuk. Nme'juinu'skwaq elmi-kwetapietaq samqwan-iktuk. Al-kiwto'qi'kwe'k tetuji wlta'sit apaji-pqwasa'sin. Klapis app powkwitesink welikwetutk ankamatl Lo'lial. "Lo'li, mita kis-wsitawi'in, iknmultes ta'n pasik koqoey pewatmn."

Ankmayiw Lo'li kisite'k ta'n koqoey pewatk. Pewatk msikiln aqq mlkiknan aqq ksaluksin.

A'tiuewiktuatl Nme'juinu'skwal aqq apaja'sit wutank aqq aknutmuajik wenik wjit Nme'juinu'skwal aqq ta'n tel-westawiasnl. Wskwijinu'k jiksitua'titl aknutmilitl aqq welima'titl wjit ta'n tel-mlkita'lij apoqnmuan Nme'juinu'skwal aqq weja'tekemkek mekite'lmut aqq maqite'lmut.

tugging at the logs with all of his heart, and suddenly the logs begin to move. He tugs and tugs and they slide right into the water! The mermaid dives in below the waves. She is swimming around, swimming around, glad to be back in the water of her life. After a little while she comes back up and looks at Loli, smiling. "You have saved my life, Loli, I'll grant you whatever wish you want."

Well, Loli doesn't have to think much about what his wish is. He wishes to be big and strong and well liked.

He says goodbye to the mermaid, and walks back to his community where he tells the story of the mermaid and how he has saved her. People come all around him to listen to his story and they praise him for his bravery and his willingness to help the mermaid and from that day on he is big and strong and well loved.

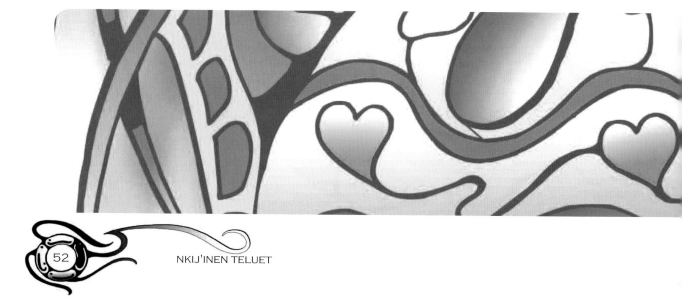

E'pijik wesku'tmi'tij tetuji-keknue'k tetpaqatalumk ta'n tujiw eskmaqtman kulaman e'pit aqq wunijan wle'taq aqq e'pit kisi-nuseskwetew kis-we'jitaq. Wesku'tmi'tij wi'n. Wi'n na etek waqn'tew-iktuk, aklasie'w-iktuk teluisik bone marrow. Wejkwa'taqnik keknue'ksip e'pit msitmn tepiaq wi'n teli-pkiji-skmaqtmaj. "Kiskuk kejitu'k wi'n waju'aq koqoey welapetmumk, staqa nike' 'iron', na'sik ki's sa'q kukmijinaqi'k kejitu'tip na." Aji-kisikuwultite'wk e'pijik mikwite'tmi'tij eskmaqtma'titijek msit wen petkitkis wi'n. Wkwijl telimtl, "Ne'wt keji'sk wen wutank eskmalt mijua'ji'j na mawte'multaq waqn'tal aqq wi'n aqq pkisitutaq na'kwek aqq tepkik. Weja'tu'tij wi'n apli'kmujk aqq pilue'k waisisk." Weskewo'ltijik ta'n tujiw Sali'j Wkiju'eml aknutk, "Jijuaqa na siwtmap wi'n kisna mu weskewite'tmu mita mu weleyiw, na'sik kejituap kikmanaq sespete'lmuksiekik, ni'n aqq nijanl, na ki'kattmap aqq welta'suatmap wen pekisituij."

The women together know the importance of eating healthily while pregnant. To care for the woman, to care for the baby, to provide the body with the nutrients to sustain the woman through the birth and to make milk to feed the baby. They talk about Wi'n. Wi'n is the Mi'kmaw name for bone marrow. They tell her that traditionally it was important for pregnant women to have Wi'n. "We know from modern knowledge that it is very high in nutrients like iron, but this was something that our grandmothers and great grandmothers have known for a long time." The older women remember that when they were pregnant, Wi'n would come from all over the community. Her Mother tells her, "Once the community knew you were pregnant, they would keep the bones and the marrow and come from across the road to give it to you, even early in the morning and late at night. It could be marrow from rabbits or anything." They all laugh when her Grandmother remembers that. "I didn't always want to eat it, when I was pregnant and maybe not feeling so good, but it was given to me by the community who cared for me and my baby so I always took it and was grateful for it."

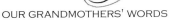

 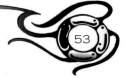

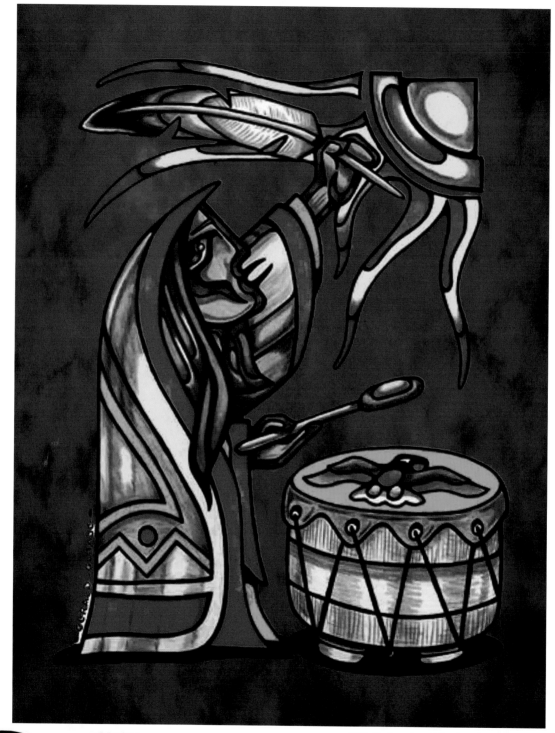

Welalin by Gerald Gloade (undated)

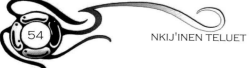

*P*emi-aji- wjuowk ika'q we'jitan, Sali'j poqji-pipanikesit, "Tala'sites net we'jitayan Kiju'?"

Kiju' telimatl, "Kesi-aji-pilua'sikip koqoey ni'n nutqweyanek. Eyki*p*nik e'pijik wutank nuji-npitaqatijik kisna nuji-apoqnmua'tipnik e'pijik we'jita'tilij. Wikumupnik ta'n tujiw e'pit ketu' we'jitaj. Aqq elp kti*k*ik e'pijik pejita'pnik naji-apoqnmua'tinew. E'pijik ta'n ki's we'jita'tijik pasi*k* asite'lmupnik i'mu'tinew wen we'jitat, aqq elp eskmaqtmaj wen asite'lmaten i'mn kulaman kisi-kina'masitew na't koqoey ke'sk mna'q nekm we'jitaq. Kkijinuaq na nuji-npiteketaq aqq i' wije'wki*p*naq naji-apoqnmuatl e'pitl we'jitalij."

"Eymu'si*p* mijua'ji'j weskwijinuit?"

Kiju' weskewe'k teluet, "E'e kaqi'sk. Aqq elp kaqi'sk we'jitay! Mu nuta'nuk sespeta'sin. Lita'suate'n ktinin aqq lita'sual knijan. Menaqaj maliamsin eskmaqtman aqq ala'li*j* wenik apoqnmulninew we'jitan, ma' l'pa taleywun. Melkiknan Sali'j, l'pa mukk we'kwata'siw, wla'sitew na ta'n teleyin."

*A*s the time for the birth is approaching, Sali'j asks, "What will the birth be like, Grandmother?"

"In my time," replies her Grandmother, "It was different to how it is now. We had women in the community who would be at the birth, medicine women, midwives who knew all about how to help the woman and the baby. And there were other women helping too. Only women who had children of her own could be at the birth, and maybe a woman who was pregnant so she could help and understand and so not be frightened of her own baby coming. Our mother was a medicine woman and sometimes I'd go and help her when a woman was having her baby."

"You have been there when a baby is born?"

"Yes," says Grandmother, "I have been at many births. And then at all of my own children too!" she laughs. "You don't have anything to worry about. Trust your body, trust your baby. If you look after how you are during your pregnancy and have good support to stay strong while you are bringing your baby into the world, then you will be fine. You are a strong woman, Sali'j. Do not be influenced by fear."

PAKO'SI

*K*i's sa'q, mawo'ltisni'k kniskamijinaqi'k aqq alqatmu'tisnik msit tami. Mu tatqi-qama'tu'tikl wikual tami ika'tij. Na telo'ltisni'k. Mu eplewkuta'tikisnik aqq milawsultikisnik. Weja'tu'tis wilu'ow maqamikew-iktuk aqq samqwan-iktuk.

THE MEDICINE BOY

*T*here was a time when the Mi'kmaq lived in different camps over the course of a year; a summer camp and a winter one. This Mi'kmaw community lives by the water in their summer camp. The Grand Chief lives here and has a

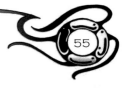

Na wla wutanji'j wikisnaq, Kji-Saqamaw aqq wtusa. Ta'nek kelu'silitl mu pasik kelu'sikaq, welmitoqsipnaq elt aqq welte'tasitaq. L'nu'k mekite'lma'tisnaq wla saqama'skwe'jaq. Msit l'pa'tu'sk welama'tisnl aqq e'tasiw pewatkis nekm kis-malie'winew na e'pite'sl. Toqa'q ika'q msit wen attikna'sit, ilajuktmi'tij wejku'aq kesik.

Na kisiku'k poqji-piltuama'titl e'pite'sl, telama'titl staqa eskmalajek mijua'ji'jl. Na kisiku'k pipanima'titl, "Wen wunijan net?" Telimaji mna'q ji'nml tekweywaql. Wunki'kuk aqq msit wen wekayik. Ta'nik sa'q wiskuala'titl telua'tijik tepias jikla'sij wutank. "Etlite'tk awsam-kelu'sit wjit kinu aqq mu ketu' kinua'tekek ta'n wenl wnijan pema'tuatl. Kespukwa'luksi'k. Jikla'sij." Na Saqamaw klapis kisa'mut essa'n wtusl. Meskita'sit pasik amujpa telimajik ji'nmuk, "Ilpalikewuk, smaqa'luk aqq nqalatoqsip knekk kisoqe'k." Kejia'titl ma' sapawsilkle mtuipuk.

E'pite's kejitoq ta'n tel-aknimut aqq kejitoq wujjl kisutmlij ta'n tla'laten, na poqtukwal ji'nmuk. Ela'la'titl knekk kisoqe'k, katu mu etenuk wkamlamunuaq skimtuk naqalanew.

beautiful daughter. She is young, only thirteen or so, and is loved by everyone. Many of the young Mi'kmaw men hope that one day, when she is older, she will choose him to be her husband.

The summer is ending and all of the community gets ready to leave the summer camp. People are busy, harvesting food in the beautiful fall weather. It is at this time that the old women, who watch everyone closely, notice that there have been certain changes in the daughter of the Chief. Although she is young and has never been seen with any man, they suspect that she is pregnant. They ask her and she says, No! There is no reason that she would be pregnant, but the old women watch her and are sure that she is carrying a child.

The question is brought to the Chief, who asks his daughter who the father is. "There is no one," she answers. But it is apparent to all that she is pregnant. Suspicions turn to rumours, which turn to spite and soon many in the community are clamouring that she be banished. "She thinks she is too good for us and won't tell us who the father is," they whisper. "She is lying to us. She should not be part of our family if she will not tell us the truth." And the Chief, torn between his responsibility of nurturing his people and his love of his daughter, is eventually persuaded to banish his daughter from the community.

With a heavy heart he tells two warriors, "Take her into the woods, and abandon her."

They all know that she is too young to survive the winter alone.

 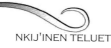

Na kisita'sijik l'tuanew wikuom aqq nu'te'lmaqn. Tujiw apaji-l'ma'tijik. Wikmawaq pempalika'tijik nqatmnew ta'n etl-qatmumk Nipk. Ma' apajita'qik nipnuk, se'kk atqatmu'titaq, atlasma'tu'tit pe'l ula tett. Kaqi-ilajulti'tij smaqita'jik.

Toqa'q aqq Kesik pemiaql, siawa'sik ta'n telo'lti'tij. Jijuaqa na na'tuen mikwite'lmatl e'pite'sl aqq ankite'tk etuk tali-tpietuknaq, katu kejitoq wkamlamunk neplitaq. Pastek wastew. Na lamikuo'mk eymu'tijik aqq epultijik kiwto'qiw nu'telmaqn aqq a'tukutijik. Etekl pitaql a'tukwaqnn, newtitpa'q kisna me' telipkijiaql. Miawipukewey wi'kipaltimk pekisitoq welta'suaqn aqq mijua'tmi'tij ta'n koqoey Kisu'lkw kis-iknmuaj.

Siwkw ika'q, ki's app poqtamkita'jik, elta'jik etlqatmumk wjit nipk. Ke'sk pemita'tij, ji'nmuk nenmi'tij ta'n eymi'tij. Eykik kikjuk etlinqala'tipnaq e'pite'saq na kimu'tuk smaqa'tijik naji-ankaptmi'tij ta'n telitpielisnaq. Ika'tij wikuom nemitu'tij ne'ipkutek nu'te'lmaqn. Etuk jel me' mimajit telita'sijik. Ejikleka'la'titl naqsun ka'qnek na nemia'titl e'pite'sl

The young woman knows what the community is saying about her, and the choice that her father has made, and she follows the two warriors into the woods. They go deep, deep into the woods, far from the summer camp, but when they get to a secluded spot the warriors agree that they cannot simply abandon her and instead help build her a wikuom and start her a fire. Then they leave her and return home to their families who are making the final preparation for leaving the summer camp. The community will not return here next summer. It will be several years before they return to the same camp as they move from camp to camp each year in order to rest the land that provides for them. With everything ready, they leave.

All the fall and all the long winter, the community continues its life. Some people think of the daughter of the Chief and wonder what happened to her, although they know in their hearts that she is dead. The blanket of winter snow lies deep on the sleeping earth. It is the time for stories to be told around the fires, some stories lasting a night, some stories lasting many nights. The Midwinter festival, the most important in the Mi'kmaw year, brings celebration and gratitude for all of the gifts of life.

In the spring the community travels to the summer camp. As they are going through the woods, the two warriors recognize that they are close to where they left the daughter of the Chief. Quietly, they leave their families to see if the wikuom is still there. They find it, still in place, with smoke coming from the top. "She is alive!" they exclaim. They elisinlitl. Na nemia'titl ne'atpa'sitl mijua'ji'jl, etl-nuseskwetl wkwijl toqo ki's neplisnaq.

Na ji'nmuk we'kwata'sijik. Kwetayakwi'titl ula mijua'ji'jl na kisita'sijik ne'pa'new. Telimtijik "Etuk ula winsitji'j ne'pata'ta wkwija toqo me' etl-nuseskwetl. Welmitoqaq aqq kelu'sitaq na e'pite'saq, ke' wutqutalanej tujiw naji-nisekenej l'pa'tuj mtasoq-iktuk."

Na kis-wutqutala'tij e'pite'sl na ela'latitl mijua'ji'jl naji-nisekenew mtasoq-iktuk, suel ika'tij na mijua'ji'j kelusa'sit, telimajik mu ne'pe'kwun. Teluet, "Mu na pisuiw petkimuksiw ula wsitqamu'k. Kji-Niskam petkimip naji-apoqnmuan L'nu'k. Pikwelk ksnukwaqn ajkneyakwi'tij L'nu'k. Peji kina'muloq L'nui-mpisun ta'n wejiaq maqamikek. Nkijjaq welmitoqaq aqq nike' kiskuk weljaqe'k Wa'so'q." Ji'nmuk pa'qalayakwi'titl tetuji apje'jilitl mijua'ji'jl kelusitl. Na tela'tekejik ta'n telimkwi'tij.

open the door of the wikuom and see the young woman lying with her back to them, near the fire. She is very still. While they are looking, frightened at what they may see, a small head appears and looks at them. It is a baby boy. He is drinking his mother's milk. But the woman is not moving and as the men get closer to her they realize that she has just died. Very recently, as there is still wood in the fire.

The warriors are frightened by the baby boy. "How can he be here?" they think. "He is trying to get milk from his poor dead mother. That is unnatural." And they decide that they must get rid of the boy. They know he will die anyway if they leave him because he would have no food and no one to care for him. First they bury the young woman and then they carry the boy out of the wikuom, toward a nearby point. They are going to throw him off the cliff and are almost there when the little boy speaks up and says, "Before you kill me, I have something to say."

The men are amazed that he is able to speak because he is only a baby, and so strong is their shock that they stop walking. The boy looks at them and continues to speak: "It was no man that brought me to my mother. I was sent here by the Great Spirit to teach native people about medicine. I was put here on Mother Earth to bring this knowledge to the Mi'kmaq, and I will teach you everything that you need."

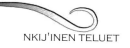

Mijua'ji'j ekina'muajik ta'n mpisunn weja'tumk saqliaqewe'l, kmu'j-iktuk, jipiskl, pisaqnatkwl aqq msit koqoey ta'n etlikwek wsitqamu'k. Poqji-wi'tikl teluisik mpisunn aqq koqoey te's nepitoq aqq ta'n tujiw kelu'kl meknmumk aqq ta'n tl-wekasiten.

Kaqi-kina'muaj L'nui-mpisunn na telimajik ela'lukwun ala kun'tew etek kikjuk qospemk. Telimajik, "Ni'n teluisi Pako'si aqq na na'te'l wji-we'ji'toqsip elmiaq nuta'yoq jikla'tulninew ksnukwaqn." Na ji'nmuk pa'qalayikik aqq wesku'tmi'tij ta'n koqoey l'pa'tuj kis-kina'muaj na kiwasklapa'tijik ankamanew na'sik ki's keska'silitaq ewne'k-iktuk. Na elma'tijik naji-kinua'tua'tij wikmawaq aqq saqmawl ta'n koqoey kis-kina'mujik. Saqamaw ti meskimut aqq meskita'sit ta'n kis-tla'laj wunijanaq. Nike' msit kejitu'tij ula e'pite'saq iknmuajek mimajuaqnmek wikmaq kulaman weskuntaq l'nui-mpisun. Na wtapekiaqnmuaq aqq wi'kipaltimkl muwala'tijik epite'sl aqq wunijan aqq siawa'tu'tij ta'n koqoey kis-kina'makwi'tipn kulaman wlo'ltitaq wtininuaq aqq ta'n telita'sulti'tij aqq teli-ktlamsitasulti'tij.

So the boy teaches the two warriors all about the medicine found in plants, in trees, in fungi, in moss, in all of the living parts of the woods and the streams, the trees and the shore. He tells them which medicine they need for each ailment, how to pick the medicine and how to prepare it. He tells them where the plant lives and what time of the season it can be picked.

When he has finished sharing all of the information, the boy says, "You don't have to get rid of me. You can set me down on this rock just here." The warriors put the boy down, amazed at all he had told them. They are talking about what they have learned and when they look down at the rock, they see that the boy is nowhere to be seen. He is gone; he has disappeared. With all of their new knowledge the men go back to their families and tell the Chief everything that happened. The Chief is very humbled by all that has passed, and saddened at how he treated his daughter. He, and all of the people, recognize that the young woman has sacrificed her life in order to bring to them the great gift of the knowledge of medicine. In their songs and feasts, the young woman and the medicine boy are thanked and since that time the Mi'kmaq have great knowledge of using medicine from the natural world to stay healthy in mind, body and spirit.

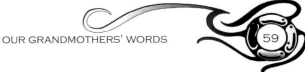

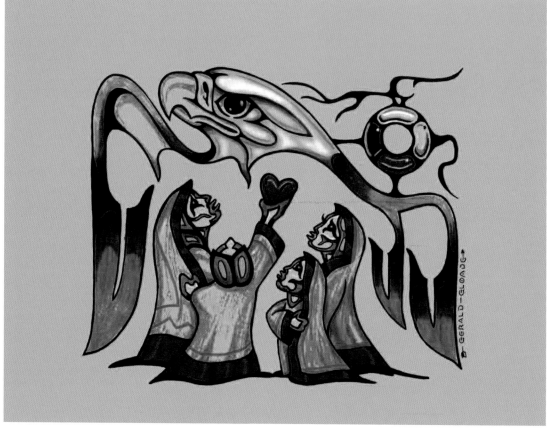

Heart of Kitpu's Home by Gerald Gloade (undated)

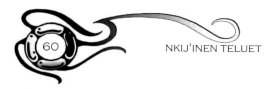

Etawaqsewut Pisaqnatkwe'j

Sali'j mikwite'tk ta'n kis-tlimsipnl Wkiju'eml ta'n tujiw naji-we'jitat. Mu we'kwata'sik. Kejitoq ta'n tela'sit wen we'jitaj. Kina'maqn weja'tuaj Wkjijl, Wjiku'eml, Wkekkunitl aqq wsukwisk ta'n nekmow tel-kina'mupnik wejkwa'taqnik. Melkiknat, melkita't aqq weli-apoqnmut. Aqq nkutey wjit wji'numuml, nekm elp kisiku'k kis-kina'majik aqq kiskaje'k menaqaj kisikwenan wunijan. Sankewo'ltijik aqq mu pekije'nuk we'jitajik e'pite'ji'jl. Sali'j aqq wji'numuml welqatkik aqq welta'sijik, Sali'j sekkapjitl wunijan wkamulamunk.

Welta'suaqn, msit wen welqatk. E'pite'ji'j we'jitamk, l'uiknek enkatiknn jel asukom teli-ksikulk. "Awsma weli-msikilk!" telua'tijik wikmaq. Maw-tmk piskwa'lujik Kiju'aq naji-ankamanew mijua'ji'jl. Kiju' ta'n wetapeksijik Muinaq nikan-piskwa't, ke'kutoqja'latl Sali'jal, menaqaj iloqama'titl mijua'ji'jl.

A blessing for the newborn

Sali'j remembers all of the Grandmothers' words as her contractions start and the time comes for her baby to be born. She does not fear. She has good knowledge about what the birth will be like. The stories of her mother and her Grandmother, her Godmother and her aunts, the stories passed down to her generation after generation have created a web of knowing around her. She is safe, she is strong, she is supported. And it is the same for her husband. He has been nurtured during the months by the Elder men in his life and is ready to be a caring parent. Together, the three of them have a peaceful birth and within only a few hours Sali'j and her husband are sitting, tired and delighted, while Sali'j holds her newborn daughter close to her heart.

The corridors are buzzing with joy and excitement. A baby girl! A baby girl! 7lbs 6oz. "A good size," they say. First to come into the room are the Grandmothers. One of them, the Clan Mother of the Bear Clan, steps forward, hugging Sali'j as they smile at the baby.

 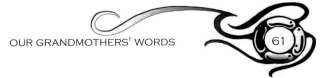

Sama'tuat mijua'ji'jl wunji kikjuk wpukwik tujiw teluet
L'nu-iktuk,

"Etawey msɨt koqoey nemitu'n klu'ktn. Ajipjulul
kepmite'tm msɨt Niskam wkisitaqnn."

Tujiw sama'tuatl wsituaqnn, teluet "Etawey msɨt
koqoey nutmn klu'ktn. Ajipjulul mu nutmn koqoey ta'n
askayulis."

Sama'tuat wtun, "Etawey msɨt koqoey teluen klu'ktn.
Ajipjulul wliman wenik te's kelusa'sin."

Sama'tuatl mijua'ji'jl wpitnn. "Etawey ula kpitnn
we'wm apoqnmajik ewle'juanu'k. Ajipjulul ne'kaw
maliaman wenik aqq wla'teken teli-pkitawsin."

Tujiw sama'tuatl mijua'ji'jl wkwatl, "Etawey ne'kaw
kkatl wije'wmnew kelu'k awti aqq koqqwaja'taqn-iktuk
la'lulin."

Ktɨkik e'pijik elp etawaqsewa'titl mijua'ji'jl tujiw Sali'j
wji'numuml ela'tuatl wkwijl pile'l wtusual kulaman Sali'j
kisi-atlasmitew kijka'.

Speaking in Mi'kmaw, she touches the little girl's head near her eyes, and blesses the newborn.

"May everything you see be good. May you appreciate all of creation."

The Grandmother touches the baby's ears.

"May everything you hear be for the goodness of all things, may you never be bothered by hearing bad things."

She touches her mouth. "May everything that you say be for the goodness of all things. May you speak only kind words."

Next she touches the baby's hands.

"I hope these stretch out to help the needy. May they take care of other people and do good for all of your life."

Finally she rests her hands on the little girl's legs. "May your feet always be on the right path, walking toward goodness."

The other women in the room add their prayers to the blessing and as her husband takes his daughter to show his mother, Sali'j relaxes to get some much-needed sleep.

KEPME'KL MI'KMAWE'L KINA'MATNEWE'L
L'uiknek te'sikl iknmakwemkl pemawsimk
aqq l'uiknek te'sikl saputa'simkl

Kesalt Kisu'lkw – Mjijamijuey
Kesalt Kkij – Mimajuaqney
Kitk mu kaqianukl

Wape'k na wjit kisiku'k aqq mijua'ji'jk mna'q l' uiknek tewijo'lti'k aqq elp wjit Oqwatnuk

Ta'n tujiw wen kaqi-ala'toq iknmakwemkl na telui'tut kisiku.

Mimajuaqn pilua'sik te's l' uiknek te'sipunqekl pemiaq

Maqtewe'k na wjit. Tke'snuk aqq wjit mjijaqamijuey.

Mekwe'k na wjit Wejkwapniaq, piley na'kwek aqq Wjipenuk

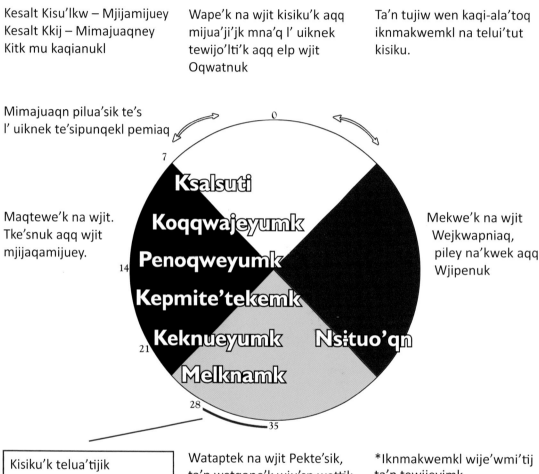

Kisiku'k telua'tijik ketlamsitasimk poqji-welnenmn na tujiw (28-35)

Wataptek na wjit Pekte'sik, ta'n wetqane'k wju'sn wettik. Melkiknewa'toq mimajuaqn

*Iknmakwemkl wije'wmi'tij ta'n tewijeyimk.

Kisiku'k ketlamsitmi'tij kisi-apaja'simk l' uiknek tewijeyumk.
Na tujiw pasik mimajuaqney kiwaska'sik. *Apaji-mijua ji'ju'en*

Apaji (preverb) – repeat, go back again. Mijua'ji'j (root word) – child under 7
U'en (inflection) – in the process of, to be, state of being

By Murdena Marshall
Graphics by Thomas Johnson
With Kristy Read